"A timely book for teachers and other school personnel working with children experiencing trauma. It's become clear that school staff need training in identifying their own signs of burnout and compassion fatigue as well as understanding and developing resiliency skills. At a time when more and more teachers are leaving the profession due to their own personal issues and job dissatisfaction, Alison DuBois and Molly Mistretta do an excellent job of describing self-efficacy and resilience and the role they play in being a highly successful educator."

—Patricia A. Markos, Ph.D., director,
Institute for Professional Studies in Education

"Teachers enter the profession to make a difference in the lives of their students, but that same deep caring and empathy can be their impetus to leave the classroom. The authors help teachers recognize the symptoms of burnout and compassion fatigue, and provide them with practical strategies for effectively dealing with stressful situations in the classroom. This is an important book for all teachers, especially those who teach in high-poverty districts."

—Faye Snodgress, executive director, Kappa Delta Pi

OVERCOMING BURNOUT AND COMPASSION FATIGUE IN SCHOOLS

This book examines the cumulative effects of working with high trauma populations as they pertain to education settings. This text incorporates current research, anecdotal stories, and workbook pages so that practitioners are properly informed on how to identify and employ protective practices when it comes to burnout and compassion fatigue.

Educators rarely receive training that prepares them for working with children and youth who are the victims of neglect, abuse, poverty, and loss. Education professionals who are already overburdened with an overwhelming amount of job-related tasks can find themselves depleted due to their care and concern for their most vulnerable students. As a result, educators experience the physical and emotional symptoms of burnout and compassion fatigue. Appropriate for both young and experienced educators, this important text provides a clear and concise approach to the topic of burnout and compassion fatigue that engages the reader in a journey of self-reflection, highlighting potential signs and symptoms of burnout, as well as examining how the school environment and individual characteristics might collide to put educators at risk.

Most importantly, this book provides guidance and resources to assist educators in implementing both individual and organizational practices that promote long-term resilience and self-care. To be their most effective, educators must be able to care for themselves while also caring for their students.

Alison L. DuBois, Ph.D., Director of the Graduate School, Westminster College, PA. For the past 23 years, Dr. DuBois, an Associate Professor of Education & Counseling, has been working with children and adolescents across a number of environments ranging from therapeutic to educational.

Molly A. Mistretta, Ph.D., Assistant Professor, Department of Counseling and Development, Slippery Rock University, PA. Dr. Mistretta's academic career has focused on preparing students and new professionals for a variety of roles within educational settings, from kindergarten through higher education.

OVERCOMING BURNOUT AND COMPASSION FATIGUE IN SCHOOLS

A Guide for Counselors, Administrators, and Educators

Alison L. DuBois and Molly A. Mistretta

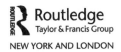

Routledge
Taylor & Francis Group

NEW YORK AND LONDON

First published 2020
by Routledge
52 Vanderbilt Avenue, New York, NY 10017

and by Routledge
2 Park Square, Milton Park, Abingdon, Oxon OX14 4RN

*Routledge is an imprint of the Taylor & Francis Group, an informa
business*

British Library Cataloguing-in-Publication Data
A catalogue record for this book is available from the British Library

Library of Congress Cataloging-in-Publication Data
Names: DuBois, Alison L., author. | Mistretta, Molly (Molly A.), author.
Title: Overcoming burnout and compassion fatigue in schools :
a guide for counselors, administrators and educators /
Alison L. DuBois and Molly A. Mistretta.
Description: Abingdon, Oxon ; New York, NY : Routledge, 2020. |
Includes bibliographical references and index.
Identifiers: LCCN 2019028309 (print) | LCCN 2019028310 (ebook) |
ISBN 9781138492646 (hardback) | ISBN 9781138492653 (paperback) |
ISBN 9781351030021 (ebook)
Subjects: LCSH: Teachers–Job stress. | Burn out(Psychology)—
Prevention. | Secondary traumatic stress—Prevention. | Teaching—
Psychological aspects.
Classification: LCC LB2840.2 .D83 2020 (print) | LCC LB2840.2
(ebook) | DDC 371.10019—dc23
LC record available at https://lccn.loc.gov/2019028309
LC ebook record available at https://lccn.loc.gov/2019028310

ISBN: 978-1-138-49264-6 (hbk)
ISBN: 978-1-138-49265-3 (pbk)
ISBN: 978-1-351-03002-1 (ebk)

Typeset in Baskerville
by codeMantra

CONTENTS

FIGURES

TABLES

1

INTRODUCTION

Education is a social process. Education is growth. Education is not a preparation for life; education is life itself.

John Dewey

Come and be a Part of the Tribe!

Humans are social beings driven by our desire to connect with one another. Child-rearing involves using a number of tools: empathy and compassion being arguably the most important. Effective educators connect with the children in care in myriad ways. Strong attachments form as they scaffold information to meet each child's developmental level in an effort to help the child make meaning of his world. Child development is an ongoing, dynamic process reliant on positive adult exchanges fostered in early childhood. Children today face multiple adversities and carry this "load" to school. Teachers, school counselors, and administrators rarely acknowledge the toll of helping children through these difficulties. Educators especially become protective of the children in their care, especially when the child's safety is compromised. The feeling of helplessness can lead professionals to despair.

Emotional togetherness, along with a passion for working with children, helps the teacher to genuinely be there—not just to be present, but to be wholly available on emotional, cognitive, and physical levels—and therefore capable of coming to genuinely understand and appropriately engage with the child. This genuine understanding and engagement is important for all children, but especially children who have experienced trauma.

(Lucas, 2007–2008, p. 88)

The Wild, Wacky World of Education

Applicants wanted. A bachelor's degree or higher is required. Applicants must be willing to work beyond the regularly contracted day. Strong communication skills are a must as applicants will have to interface with a dizzying array of individuals including but not limited to colleagues, administrators, a large caseload, and the general populace who possess little understanding or even respect for the nature of the job. Flexibility is also a must, as the demands of the job can change rapidly and with little warning. Applicants must also be willing to accept lower wages than other professionals with a bachelor's degree. Teaching sounds glamorous, right? What draws us to the field of education? I have worked as or alongside teachers for over 20 years and I have heard one response over and over from individuals entering the teaching profession: it is simply their calling to make a difference in a child's life. Teaching children with complex issues can create complex problems for us as professionals, however. As a first-year teacher, almost 25 years ago, I discovered quickly that on any given day I functioned as a teacher, counselor, nurse, cheerleader—you get the idea. As my students came to school grappling with some serious trauma, I had to learn how to help them cope with what they were experiencing so that some classroom learning could take place. I found that I was wholly ill-equipped to handle the task. Nothing in my teacher training program even addressed the topic of trauma, let alone how to address the complex thoughts and feelings generated as a result of creating a safe space for my students. Years later, after much additional schooling (M.A. and Ph.D. in Counseling), I realized that I did not cope well. I also began to identify signs of secondary trauma in my staff, who had little to no training in this area either. I not only was witnessing the personal, psychic toll this secondary trauma had on my staff, I could clearly see how this affected their functioning—and ultimately their efficacy—in the classroom. The task became clear: school personnel needed training in accurately identifying the signs of burnout and compassion fatigue, in addition to resiliency skill development.

The Evolution of Education:
The Good, the Bad, and the Ugly

At the beginning of the nineteenth century, an emphasis on moral and value development in the curriculum occurred, changing the educational pedagogy landscape. Gender bias was also prevalent with society largely believing that *rational* attributes were ascribed to men and *emotional* attributes were largely possessed by women. As a result, men "administrated" and women "taught." By the end of the century, industrialization expanded urban areas, contributing to a number of social issues. A fear began to take hold that these urban areas would experience a loss of community and social control, an increase in crime, and poverty (Spring, 2001). After almost of century of instructional practices focusing entirely on morals/values education—taught almost solely by women—pressure was put on educational institutions to be a "cure all" for society's ills. Spring states, "School was considered a logical institution to prevent these problems by providing social services, teaching new behaviors, and creating a community center" for children and adults in an effort to "reduce (neighborhood) delinquency" (2001, p. 229). Teachers saw their roles and responsibilities shift to now expanding the professional work environment beyond the school setting and interfacing with various community-based systems. Fast forward 60-plus years and urban decay and poverty were still prevalent in society. In 1963, Robert Heller presented a report *The Problem with Poverty in America*, and once again, the conclusion was made that education could be a major factor in "uprooting the culture of poverty" (Spring, 2001, p. 372) and it was stated that schools must play an even *larger* role in education, starting with preschool-aged children. Today, there are even a number of programs that target birth through age five to provide intervention early and often to reduce risk factors in dysfunctional home environments that negatively impact child development. Educators are interfacing daily with children who are suffering the deleterious effects of trauma, poverty, and poor parenting practices. As a result of this historical educational evolution, educators are struggling daily with a multitude of issues ranging from large class sizes/caseloads to meeting the wide range of educational needs in the classroom to the management of difficult behaviors. No wonder we approach our students exhausted and overwhelmed. To quote Crash Davis in the movie *Bull Durham*, "We're dealing with a lot of sh—."

The Role of Trauma in Teacher Attrition

There are many factors that influence teacher attrition. First are the individual dispositions, skills, and abilities that influence how well educators respond to the school environment, such as the number of students served and diversity of students' learning needs. Teachers are also affected by the quality of their immediate environment and the variety of interactions that occur each day, including student to teacher, teacher to para-professional, teacher to teacher, and teacher to administrator. Other attrition factors include the availability and quality of administrative and collegial support, teachers' perceptions of their roles and responsibilities, and opportunities for further training (Miller, Brownell, & Smith, 1999).

A teacher's work experience is also affected by decision-making that significantly influences a teacher's day-to-day responsibilities (Miller, Brownell, & Smith, 1999). Often, teachers have little control over important decisions that impact the classroom or the students. This lack of decision-making making control can have drastic effects on the teacher's perceived efficacy. The more positively a teacher perceives their teaching efficacy, the more likely he or she will demonstrate satisfaction with the profession and display resiliency when facing negative situations (Miller, Brownell, & Smith, 1999).

Decisions made at the state and early childhood organizational levels often involve changes and increases in paperwork (Miller, Brownell, & Smith, 1999). Salary, job benefits, and service delivery systems also influence teacher satisfaction (Miller, Brownell, & Smith, 1999). The socio-economic levels and diversity of the community also influence the teaching environment (Brownell & Smith, 1993). These are manifested in cultural beliefs, school budgetary issues, and school board decisions that affect teachers (Brownell & Smith, 1993).

Educators often experience a number of implicit and explicit demands from their work environment compelling them to act in specific ways (Lazarus, 1995). As a result of the need to "fit in," or be perceived by co-workers and supervisors as "competent," some behaviors can interfere with the coping process. For example, an educator with too heavy a caseload may eliminate some of the burden making others perceive him or her as incompetent or ineffective in executing the responsibilities of their job.

All of these factors associated with educator attrition have a direct impact on the educational process occurring within the classroom. When teachers are working in low socio-economic, culturally diverse schools with children frequently immersed in chaos and potentially traumatizing situations, the personal toll can be significant. Teachers face a multitude of sociological factors, including but not limited to a significant rise in single parent households, child abuse, poverty, and diverse systemic needs. For an educator, the management for all of these variables and systems can be quite overwhelming and stressful.

The attrition literature has linked teacher attrition and/ or job dissatisfaction to several key areas. Research has found that young, inexperienced special educators are twice as likely to leave the profession as compared to their more experienced colleagues (Singer, 1993; Billingsley, 2004). Older teachers tend to leave the profession as a result of retirement (Billingsley, 2004). Cole's (1992) research found that personal characteristics have a direct impact on a teacher's professional practice, the work environment, and the relationships that she develops with colleagues. All of these factors can contribute to whether the teacher will remain in the field or leave it. The notion of burnout is frequently referenced in the attrition literature. It is usually referred to as "emotional exhaustion" or a sense of "depersonalization" in relation to the teacher's work efficacy.

Beating the Pitfall of Teacher Attrition

Teachers' positive perceptions of self-efficacy have been shown to be positively connected to whether or not they will stay in the field. Teachers who are self-confident in their abilities believe they make a greater impact on the children they teach, which in turn leads to intrinsic rewards or feelings of compassion satisfaction for doing their job. When questioned during the individual interviews about how they viewed their effectiveness in the classroom, they responded,

> *I always thought I was a pretty effective teacher ... I could see my kids learn ... I learned to appreciate the small things, the small gains, rather than the big, huge "Oh my God, I taught them all their letters and numbers" ... I think you have to look at the small steps ... That was always the exciting part for me, the small steps.*
>
> *I think so [that I'm a good teacher]. I really think that I've seen so many changes in children by the time they leave ... I think we feel really good when they leave that we've done something for them.*
>
> *I'm pretty confident in the classroom. The first year teaching, I certainly wasn't. But with the help of other people to help build your confidence ... you feel like you are a better teacher.*

Stamm (2002) has found in her research that individuals possess an instinctual ability to self-protect when confronted with trauma material. Resilience enables a person to confront life's adversities by developing positive patterns of behavioral responses. Resilience is a major component of compassion satisfaction. Colleague and administrative support (Billingsley, 2004; Stamm, 2002) and positive school climate and opportunities for additional training (Billingsley, 2004) all contribute to a teacher's ability to preserve and develop constructive coping mechanisms when faced with traumatic stressors.

What Do You Do with the Hurt That You Feel?

Teacher training programs focus almost entirely on curriculum and instructional teaching methods, behavior management, and testing and assessment practices. The reality is that once pre-service teachers are in a school setting, they are faced with a different set of roles and responsibilities they have not been prepared to face. Educators must employ a number of coping mechanisms to deal with myriad facets of their job. The pressure of handling various administrative roles and responsibilities—including large caseloads, frequently changing paperwork requirements, standardized test scores often linked to teacher evaluation, and most importantly, meeting the developmental and educational needs of the children in their care—can be overwhelming. Taking some deep, cleansing breaths is in order! Research has demonstrated that personnel with prior training and experience are better able to implement self-care strategies, thereby reducing the risk of burnout and compassion fatigue (Jaycox et al., 2007). Each day educators face mounting pressure to meet learning objectives and demonstrate student progress. Compassion fatigue can affect an individual cognitively, emotionally, behaviorally, and spiritually (Figley, 2002).

This book seeks to de-mystify the concepts surrounding childhood trauma and provide educators with a toolkit to employ when their "load" becomes too great. We will discuss a theoretical framework that explains the impact of trauma and the effect of systems on children and educators. Practical strategies to implement in times of distress will also be presented.

How to Use This Book

We want you to be able to implement authentic, lasting changes to your personal and professional work lives. This book was written to be a user-friendly, interactive, engaging tool to help practitioners learn the signs and symptoms of burnout, compassion fatigue, and compassion satisfaction, in addition to implementing easy strategies that help enable you to reduce your risk of developing burnout and/or compassion fatigue. The ultimate goal is to develop healthy habits that develop into stronger resiliency skills—making you a more effective, engaging educator that continues to find purpose and meaning professionally.

This book can be used in a number of ways: individually; as part of an on-going professional development training at staff meetings; during de-briefing sessions with administrators; in small groups composed of mentors/mentees. We encourage you to set time aside each week to review a chapter, answer the reflection questions meaningfully and discuss with peers thoughtfully, and try the strategies consistently.

Burnout and compassion fatigue are not a death sentence. By choosing this book, you have taken the first step in investing in a healthier you. To use the analogy, "You have to put your oxygen mask on first before helping the child sitting next you!" By adopting the appropriate self-care strategies, you can not only thrive—but *flourish*—despite a challenging educational environment. Take some deep, cleansing breaths … Let's begin!

References

Billingsley, B. S. (2004). Special education teacher retention and attrition: A critical analysis of the research literature. *The Journal of Special Education, 38*(1), 39–55.

Brownell, M. T., & Smith, S. W. (1993). Understanding special education teacher attrition: A conceptual model and implications for teacher educators. *Teacher Education and Special Education, 16*(3), 270–282.

Burg, M., & Shelton, R. (1988). *Bull Durham.* USA: The Mount Company

Cole, A. L. (1992). Teacher development in the work place: Rethinking the appropriation of professional relationships. *Teachers College Record, 94*(2), 365–381.

Figley, C. R. (Ed.) (2002). *Treating compassion fatigue* (1st ed.). New York, NY: Brunner-Routledge.

Jaycox, L. H., Tanielian, T. L., Sharma, P., Morse, L., Clum, G., & Stein, B. D. (2007). Schools' mental health responses after Hurricane Katrina and Rita. *Psychiatric Services, 58*(10), 1339–1343.

Lazarus, R. S. (1995). Psychological stress in the workplace. In R. Crandall & P. L. Perrewé (Eds.), *Occupational stress: A handbook* (pp. 3–14). Washington, DC: Taylor Francis.

Lucas, L. (2007–2008). The of attachment: you have to put a little wedge in there. *Childhood Education, 84*(2), 85–91.

Miller, M. D., Brownell, M. T., & Smith, S. W. (1999). Factors that predict teachers staying in, leaving, or transferring from the special education classroom. *Exceptional Children, 65*(2), 201–218.

Singer, J. D. (1993). Once is not enough: Former special educators who return to teaching. *Exceptional Children, 60*(1), 58–72.

Spring, J. (2001). *The American school* (5th ed.). Boston, MA: McGraw Hill.

Stamm, B. (2002). Measuring compassion satisfaction as well as fatigue: Developmental history of the compassion fatigue and satisfaction test. In C. R. Figley (Ed.), *Treating Compassion Fatigue* (pp. 107–119). New York: Brunner/Mazel.

2

THE DEVELOPMENTAL
IMPACT OF TRAUMA

*To endure is the first thing a child ought to learn, and that which
he will have the most need to know.*

Jean-Jacques Rousseau

Today's modern families are dealing with a variety of stressors that
are complex and wide-ranging in nature. We spend an inordinate
amount of time engaging in media per day allowing our mental
load to become too great. These stressors can also play a significant
role in a child's development. As a result, educators are challenged
daily to meet myriad needs of their students that go far beyond the
curriculum. Over time, an emotional toll is experienced by these
professionals. The equation is simple, if you improve your overall
quality of life, you will be far more effective and responsive when
dealing with complicated student needs. When educators first start
working in the field, they have a set of expectations based on their
pre-service training and education. Then, they meet their students
and are now a full-fledged member of the work environment,
which is often guided by different principles—thereby not align-
ing with their pre-conceived expectations and creating a cognitive
dis-connect (Riley, San Juan, Klinker, & Ramminger, 2008).

This chapter will explore two angles of trauma: first, how it impacts a child developmentally; and second, how many educators
who have their own personal trauma histories can be affected
personally and professionally.

Connections, Connections, Connections

Attachment and exploration are critical developmental behaviors that a young child will instinctively demonstrate. A child's ability to form strong attachments allows him to develop trust and a sense of safety, enabling him to explore the world around him and gain new knowledge from these experiences. Attachments begin first with parents, then move to teachers. Nurturing, effective parenting helps assuage a child's anxieties—resulting in opportunities for the child to take risks, learn, and grow. Positive feelings and emotions between caregiver and child also form the backbone of a child's ability to develop empathy and social cognition (Decety & Meyer, 2008).

> *All actions are based on the ground the person happens to stand upon. The firmness of his actions and the clearness of his decision depend largely on the stability of this "ground," although he himself may not even be aware of its nature.*
>
> (Lewin, 1948, p. 148)

Strong attachments in the home environment enable children to generalize those skills to other environments, like school. Securely attached preschoolers demonstrate increased compliance, more control over emotional regulation, a natural curiosity to explore their environment more, a stronger sense of self and internal locus of control, the ability to delay gratification, stronger attending skills, solid peer relationships, and the ability to accept comfort when distressed (Riley et al., 2008; Pollack, 2005; Goleman, 2005; Decety & Meyer, 2008). Research has found that children who have formed positive, secure attachments demonstrate higher performance levels in assessments requiring cognitive skills through age 17 (Jacobsen, Edelstein, & Hofmann, 1994).

Roughly one in five children (Riley et al., 2008) do not have a secure relationship with their parents or caregivers. Disrupted attachments can lead to harm in all developmental areas (Bloom & Sreedhar, 2008). Possessing the skill to accurately process one's own and subsequently a parent's emotional state is the foundation of empathy.

Human beings are social creatures with a need to fit in and belong. Our emotional intelligence, that is, our ability to connect and relate effectively with others, is a critical indicator in our success later in life. Being able to effectively read (in the sense of reacting and understanding) others' emotions helps us make better predictions about other people's emotional states (Decety & Meyer, 2008).

Children Do Not Grow Up in a Vacuum

Lewin (1948) eschewed a developmental, as opposed to research, perspective on human psychology. He posited that children resided in the middle of several "spheres," which represented different contexts or environments that were constantly interacting with one another as the child developed. Lewin believed that the space is not physical but psychological. Features in these structures could include the movement towards a goal, connection between people across settings, and various forces interacting over a larger picture. This scholarship created the trajectory for Urie Bronfenbrenner's work.

In Bronfenbrenner's Bioecological Model of Human Development, the child sits in the middle of his system. Environmental conditions consist mainly of the interactions the child engages in daily (Bronfenbrenner, 2005). All of the child's actions and interactions with people in addition to environmental factors encompass these processes. Vygotsky (1978) states that "psychological analysis of objects should be contrasted with the analysis of processes, which requires a dynamic display of the main points making up the processes' history" (p. 60). These processes are based on the child's perception of their experiences of living in that environment (Bronfenbrenner, 2005). The interactions must occur frequently and consistently over time in the child's immediate environment in order to be considered proximal processes. Bronfenbrenner (2005) posits that children must continually have opportunities to engage in increasingly complex activities on a regular basis to develop in all areas. He also asserts that caregiver attachment is a critical element enabling children to engage with their environment so that they grow and develop.

The Microsystem, or the child's "inner circle," consists of all of the child's caregivers, and his various settings (home, school, community), such as the library or playground. All of the experiences and connections between two or more of these settings have a direct influence and are considered in the Mesosystem. These interactions can include home and school, daycare center and school, etc. (Bronfenbrenner, 2005). When one setting does not encompass the child on a regular basis, but does have the capacity to influence interactions/processes in the children's immediate setting, the Exosystem becomes involved. For example, children typically do not go to work with their parents, but a mother being reprimanded by her supervisor, thereby having a difficult day at work, can translate into how she parents her child once at home. The Macrosystem includes all previous systems and adds the child's exposure to the family's belief systems, involvement with social organizations, and societal culture at large (Bronfenbrenner, 2005). The last piece to the model includes the Chronosystem, which examines how all of these interactions affect the child's development over time. For example, the effects of poverty on a child who is exposed to housing or food insecurity briefly (i.e. dad loses his job for six months) as compared to a child living in inter-generational poverty yield far different developmental outcomes.

Childhood Maltreatment

Cicchetti and Howes (1991) found that children exposed to early environmental distress, including maltreatment, deprivation, poverty, and trauma are more at risk for delays in social, emotional, and behavioral areas, which can result in problems later in life. Poverty wreaks significant and disastrous effects on a child's development. Their health and subsequent

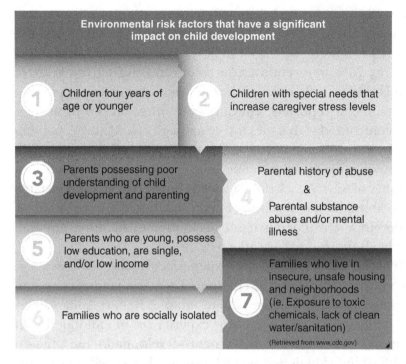

Figure 2.1 **Environmental risk factors that have a significant impact on child development.**

development can be compromised by poor quality living conditions and limited nutritional options (Pachter, Auinger, Palmer, & Weitzman, 2006). Families living in poverty are likely to have limited healthcare options, poor quality childcare, and schools with limited resources (Pachter et al., 2006). Children living in lower socio-economic households are more likely to be exposed to violence in addition to having changes to residence due to eviction or moving (Loseke, Gelles, & Cavanaugh, 2005; Evans, 2004). Communities that experience poverty, large matriarchal families, and high tenant turnover also pose an increased risk for child maltreatment (Coulton, Korbin, Su, & Chow, 1995). Impoverished families are also at a 40% higher risk of having a child diagnosed with a disability (Meyers, Lukemeyer, & Sneeding, 1998). According to the Children's Defense

Fund (https://www.childrensdefensefund.org/policy/policy-priorities/child-poverty), one in five children, totaling more than 13.2 million, were poor in 2016; over 45% lived in extreme poverty; 70% were children of color; and during the years of rapid brain growth, one in five children under six live in poverty. As mandated reporters, educators are often on the front lines and confronted with issues involving neglect and abuse, helping children cope and adjust through the investigative process.

Growing up in an unstable household affects children in a number of ways. A lack of basic needs ranging from food instability to abuse has far reaching, long-term consequences. All areas of development (cognitive, social-emotional, adaptive, physical, and communication) are affected.

What are adverse childhood experiences and how do they affect the neurodevelopment of children? Over the course of several decades and using a large patient sample, Robert Anda (2006) and colleagues investigated how experiences in childhood with a negative valence affected the neurodevelopment and physical health of individuals across the lifespan. They called these experiences Adverse Childhood Experiences, or ACEs, and defined them as any experience that is stressful or traumatic, such as abuse, neglect, witnessing domestic violence, or growing up with alcohol or other related substance abuse, mental illness, parental discord or crime in the home (2006). The researchers found that early traumatic childhood experiences "are a common pathway to social, emotional, and cognitive impairments that lead to increased risk of unhealthy behaviors, risk of violence or re-victimization, disease, disability, and premature mortality" (Anda et al., 2006, p. 15). In essence, ACEs affect the normal neurodevelopment of the brain and can have a long-term impact on the brain's structure and function. One of the most striking discoveries of this study was that ACEs are quite common: more than two-thirds of the participants—and there were around 18,000 participants—had experienced at least one ACE, and one or two out of every ten adults had experienced five or more ACEs. Additionally, these experiences were found to be interrelated and co-occurring; for example, a child experiencing neglect may have a parent who is an opioid user. One additional factor having an impact has to do with time. The cumulative effect of these experiences can permanently alter the brain and wreak havoc on the body (Anda et al., 2006). Neuroscientists have linked childhood maltreatment to long-term changes in several areas of the brain including the pre-frontal cortex, hippocampus, amygdala, corpus callosum, and cerebellum. Early stressors in childhood also demonstrate changes in their stress-responsive neurobiological systems, affecting emotional regulation, the processing of somatic signals, memory, arousal, and feelings of anger and aggression (Anda et al., 2006). Anda and colleagues were able to use modern medicine to prove what Vygotsky and Bronfenbrenner were claiming for decades: early positive interactions between a caregiver and child matter.

Children who have experienced maltreatment have a difficult time decoding facial expressions that depict emotions (Pollack, 2005). Deficits in empathy manifest themselves developmentally in a variety of ways: response inhibition, self-regulation, task initiation, cognitive flexibility, and goal directed persistence (Dawson & Guare, 2004; Decety & Meyer, 2008). A lack of impulse control impacts a child's ability to follow through and complete tasks (including social activities), in addition to incorporating new educational concepts into their repertoire of knowledge (Goleman, 2005). Each of these skills are critical to meeting early developmental outcomes, which then create the necessary building blocks for future academic success.

The Brain is a Cool Place

Let's breakdown how this works in the brain. Neurons (aka nerve cells) and neuroglia (the neurons' supporting cells) are the foundation of the central nervous system (Dawson & Guare, 2004). A neuron is made up of a cell body (called an axon) and its branch-like dendrites. The dendrites' job is to pick up and send signals (electrical impulses) to one another (Beckham & Leber, 1995). These electrical impulses change to a chemical one (called a neurotransmitter) as it travels from the dendrites to the axon. A synapse occurs when one chemical message passes from one neuron to another (Beckham & Leber, 1995). Because our brains are highly efficient, hard-working machines, these signals are insulated to increase their speed. This insulation is called myelin and the process of myelination begins in the earliest stages of development and carries on through a child's adolescent years (Dawson & Guare, 2004). Genetic determinants usually play a large role when the child is typically developing; however, the role of environment has been shown to have a significant impact as well.

Most researchers contend that cognitive development takes place in the frontal and pre-frontal cortex of the brain (Dawson & Guare, 2004). Through use of fMRI, scientists have determined that the prefrontal area of the brain is among the last to develop—typically in late adolescence—and houses working memory and processes information. When the cerebral cortex is typically developing, there is an even distribution of neurons (Grossman et al., 2003). Significant, detrimental effects to the cerebral cortex can occur, however, when a disruption occurs during cortical organization (Grossman et al., 2003).

Throughout the lifespan, plasticity also allows the brain to adapt to new information and situations. Plasticity, or neuroplasticity, is the brain's ability to reorganize neural pathways when an individual engages in a new experience when new skills are needed to function effectively (JFK Center for Research on Human Development, 2010). Beginning at about age two and a half, the brain begins to undergo the process of "pruning," thereby deciding what information is important to keep and what information can be discarded. Plasticity allows the brain to "prune" effectively, so that adaption to a new environment can occur. During this pruning process, experiences occurring frequently, such as proximal processes, have a strong influence and are "kept," while the brain lets go of the weaker connections (JFK Center for Research on Human Development, 2010). Grossman et al. (2003) state, the "capacity for plasticity later in life can, as a result, be positively or negatively influenced by these factors, making the brain more or less able to adapt to future demands" (p. 38).

Action ... Reaction!

When the brain encounters a traumatic stimulus, the processes that occur are quite intricate and complex. For the purposes of this chapter, a brief overview of the bio-physiological changes occurring during this process will be discussed. When a person is confronted with an experience or situation they have not yet encountered, an auditory or visual signal is first sent (by way of the thalamus) to the amygdala and hippocampus (memory storage site) and then on to the neocortex (Goleman, 2005). The amygdala, from the Greek work *almond,* is an almond-shaped cluster of interconnected structures that rests just below the limbic ring and just above the brainstem. The amygdala is crucial, as it responsible for determining the emotional valence of the event. The amygdala sends a "distress" signal to other parts of the brain—if the event is unknown or potentially threatening—triggering an emergency response hormone (CRH or Corticotrophin-releasing hormone), which readies the large muscle groups and cardiovascular system for a quick response (Goleman, 2005). Another signal is sent from the adrenal glands to release epinephrine and norepinephrine (aka adrenaline and noradrenaline) to activate other key areas in the brain that might be needed. The neo-cortex, or "thinking brain," develops a more detailed reaction to the experience and organizes the information for meaning, so that the brain can better understand the stimuli (Goleman, 2005).

The release of epinephrine and norepinephrine prepare the body for stress and activate receptors on the vagus nerve—which is responsible for sending signals to the heart (Goleman, 2005). During this whole process, the amygdala serves as a depository for emotional memory, comparing the current event with anything previously experienced. While all of this is going on, the amygdala also sends a signal to the limbic system to discharge catecholamines, epinephrine, and norepinephrine to mobilize the body for an emergency response (Goleman, 2005). The hypothalamus kicks into gear sending signals to the pituitary gland to release cortisol (aka "stress" neurotransmitter). A glitch in the system occurs when the present stimuli is minimal, but an emotional memory from the past triggers the amygdala into action. When this occurs over and over, changes in the limbic system can take place as the pituitary gland releases cortisol consistently, alerting the body over and over again to an emergency that is not really there.

When traumatic events happen early on in a child's life, various brain structures, such as the hippocampus, responsible for storing narrative memories, and the neocortex, which is the center for rational thought, can be drastically altered (Goleman, 2005). The neocortex modulates the amygdala and other limbic areas allowing for a more rational, analytic response. When a stress signal comes into the brain, the prefrontal lobes (responsible for working memory) experience neural static which then inhibits the lobes to use working memory effectively (Goleman, 2005). Consequently, emotional distress in childhood can create deficits in intellectual function and abilities (i.e. working memory, planning, organization, and metacognition), thereby inhibiting the capacity to learn new concepts. It also increases the likelihood that agitation and impulsivity, diminished capacities for self-regulation, task initiation, response inhibition, mental flexibility and persistence can occur (Dawson & Guare, 2004).

Increased cortisol levels in the brain can impair an individual in three ways: (1) it can interfere with the brain's supply of glucose; (2) it can interfere with the function of neurotransmitters, such as serotonin, norepinephrine, and dopamine; and (3) it causes an influx of calcium into brain cells which can kill them (Khalsa & Stauth, 1997), Once the brain is damaged by cortisol, the child has difficulty paying attention—resulting in poor memory retention—lowering the individual's ability to absorb information quickly and hold onto the information long term (Khalsa & Stauth, 1997). High epinephrine levels keep the child in a high state of alert, making concentration, social awareness, sleep, and attention difficult.

The deleterious effects of trauma are often the underpinnings of a child's maladjustment to all environments (school, home, community). Challenging behaviors can pose problems for caregivers, educators, school counselors, and administrators who are ill-equipped to handle the situation effectively. Children who are traumatized often have immature, underdeveloped coping mechanisms (Bloom & Sreedhar, 2008). Their schemas for making meaning, possessing hope, and having faith and a sense of purpose are still forming. They are in the process of discovering right and wrong, compassion and forbearance, punishment versus justice. All of their cognitive processes, such as decision-making, problem-solving, and acquisition of new skills are in the process of becoming. Trauma interferes with this typical development process (Bloom & Sreedhar, 2008).

Trauma's Long Reach

In a study conducted with early childhood special educators, DuBois (2010) found that all of the participants had experienced at least one ACE. Two-thirds of the participants had experienced two or more. As a result of the ACEs study, adverse childhood experiences were found to be quite common. Educators, who themselves may have experienced ACEs, are working in an environment where they are vicariously confronted with similar material. Their neuro-circuitry could be impaired due to their own early childhood experiences, and as they are exposed to daily stressors—their ability to respond constructively and effectively can be impaired. Stress and anxiety are experienced when an individual's cognitive and emotional load exceed their capacity to properly deal with the demands. Lazarus (1999) states, "If the ratio of demands to resources becomes too great, we are no longer talking about high stress but trauma" (p. 58).

Caring and Coping with Trauma

Not all individuals who experience trauma experience post-traumatic symptoms. According to Carlson (1997), there are a few critical elements that make a given experience traumatic. The event itself must be perceived by the person experiencing it as having a "severely negative valence" (Carlson, 1997, p. 28). Human beings instinctually avoid nasty experiences. If the individual is unable to avoid painful stimuli and this results in overwhelming feelings of sudden fear, the experience can be traumatizing. Timing also plays a crucial role. "The critical factor here is the amount of time between the person's awareness of a danger and the danger itself because that is the amount of time that a person has to act or to process the negative event" (Carlson, 1997, p. 31). Another essential element concerns an individual's perceived measure of control during the event. The more powerless they feels during the situation, the greater the likelihood the event will feel traumatic. The role an individual plays during the event—voluntary, involuntary, or predictable—can also affect a person's perception of the incident (Carlson, 1997). Three other important elements have to do with time. The frequency with which the event occurs, the swiftness of an individual's response to the negative stimuli in conjunction with their ability to find safety quickly can also impact a person's perception (Carlson, 1997).

So what makes an event traumatic? Green (1993) categorizes seven dimensions of trauma. These can include:

- Acts of human aggression as defined by threats to a person's physical body, intentional or unintentional, individually or collectively (i.e. neighborhood gang violence).
- Exposure to the loss of a loved one that can be sudden or violent.
- Causing serious harm to another individual.
- Natural or man-made disasters (i.e. hurricanes, school shootings, car accidents).

Self-Reflective Questions for Thoughtful Practice

This chapter examined the developmental impact of trauma, in addition to how educators with personal trauma histories can be affected both personally and professionally. Strong and early attachments matter, as well as protective factors like a supportive family and social network, access to healthcare and social services, and stability in acquiring basic needs. The questions below encourage you to analyze trauma's impact on you both personally and professionally.

1. *What are some risk factors and/or ACEs that children on your caseload experience daily?*

   _____

   _____

   _____

   _____

   _____

2. *How do these risk factors affect the children's developmental levels and/or classroom learning?*

   _____

   _____

   _____

   _____

   _____

3. *How does the brain process a traumatic event?*

   _____

   _____

   _____

   _____

   _____

4. *Examining your own history, have you experienced any ACEs/Environmental Risk Factors? If so, how did these experiences impact your development? What impact do they have in your current practice?*

_____

_____

_____

_____

5. *Have you experienced a work situation where your personal history interfered with the way you dealt with the issue? If so, what would you do differently if a similar situation occurred?*

_____

_____

_____

_____

Additional Resources

The following website has additional information on risk factors affecting child development: https://www.cdc.gov/
https://www.youtube.com/watch?v=95ovIJ3dsNk
Diltrot, J., Hamilton, L., Maughan, B., & Snowling, M. (2017). Child and environmental risk factors predicting readiness for learning in children at high risk of dyslexia. *Developmental Psychopathology, 29*(1), 235–244.

References

Anda, R. F., Felitti, V. J., Walker, J., Whitfield, C. L., Cremner, J. D., Perry, B. D., Dube, S. R., Giles, W. H. (2006). The enduring effects of abuse and related adverse experiences in childhood: A convergence of evidence from neurobiology and epidemiology. *European Archives of Psychiatry & Clinical Neurosciences, 256*(3), 174–186.

Beckham, E. E., & Leber, W. R. (1995). *Handbook of depression* (2nd ed.). New York, NY: Guilford Press.

Bloom, S. L. & Sreedhar, S. Y. (2008). The sanctuary model of trauma informed organizational change. *Reclaiming Children and Youth, 17*(3), 49–53.

Bronfenbrenner, U. (2005). *Making human beings human.* Thousand Oaks, CA: Sage Publications.

Carlson, E. (1997). *Trauma assessments: A clinician's guide.* New York, NY: The Guilford Press.

Cicchetti, D., & Howes, P. W. (1991). Developmental psychopathology in the context of the family: illustrations from the study of child maltreatment. *Canadian Journal of Behavioral Science, 23*(3), 257–281.

Coulton, C. J., Korbin, J. E., Su, M., & Chow, J. (*1995*). Community level factors and child maltreatment rates. Child Development, *66*(5), 1262–1276.

Dawson, P., & Guare, R. (2004). *Executive skills in children and adolescents.* New York, NY: The Guildford Press.

Decety, J. & Meyer, M., (2008). From emotion resonance to empathic understanding: A social developmental neuroscience account. *Development and Psychopathology, 20,* 1053–1080.

DuBois, A. L. (2010). *An inquiry of the lived experiences and contextual understandings of early childhood special educators related to children's trauma* (Doctoral dissertation). Retrieved from *https://eric.ed.gov/?id=ED522137*

Evans, G. (2004). The environment of childhood poverty. *The American Psychologist, 59*(2), 77–92.

Goleman, D. (2005). *Emotional intelligence* (2nd ed.). New York, NY: Bantam Books.

Green, A. (1993). Childhood sexual and physical abuse. In J. Wilson & B. Raphael (Eds.), *International Handbook of Traumatic Stress Syndromes,* (pp. 577–592). New York: Plenum Press.

Grossman, A. W., Churchill, J. D., McKinney, B. C., Kodish, I. M., Otte, S. L., & Greenough, W. T. (2003). Experience effects on brain development: Possible contributions to psychopathology. *Journal of Child Psychology and Psychiatry, 44*(1), 33–63.

Jacobsen, T., Edelstein, W., & Hofmann, V. (1994) A longitudinal study of the relation between representations of attachment in childhood and cognitive functioning in childhood and adolescence. *Dev Psycho, 30*(1), 112–124.

JFK Center for Research and Human Development. (2010). Retrieved on September 2, 2018 from https://vkc.mc.vanderbilt.edu/vkc/about/history/.

Khalsa, D. S. & Stauth, C. (1997). *Brain longevity.* New York, NY: Warner Books.

Lazarus, R. S. (1999). *Stress and emotion: A new synthesis.* New York, NY: Springer Publishing Co.

Lewin, K. (1948). *Resolving social conflicts.* New York, NY: Harper & Brothers.

Loseke, D., Gelles, R. & Cavanaugh, M. (Eds.) (2005). *Current controversies on family violence.* Thousand Oaks, CA: Sage.

Meyers, T., Lukemeyer, A. & Smeeding, T. (1998). The cost of caring: Childhood disability and poor families. *Social Service Review, 72,* 209–234.

Pachter, L. M., Auinger, P., Palmer, R., & Weitzman, M. (2006). Do parenting and the home environment, maternal depression, neighborhood, and chronic poverty affect child behavioral problems differently in different racial-ethnic groups? *Pediatrics, 117*(4), 1329–1338.

Pollack, S. D. (2005). Early adversity and mechanisms of plasticity: Integrating affective neuroscience with developmental approaches to psychopathology. *Development and Psychopathology, 17,* 735–752.

Riley, D. San Juan, R. R., Klinkner, J., & Ramminger, A. (2008). *Social & emotional development.* St. Paul, MN: Red Leaf Press.

Vygotsky, L. (1978). *Mind in society.* Cambridge, MA: Harvard University Press.

3

RISK FACTORS THAT CREATE THE PERFECT STORM

What Puts Me at Risk for Burnout and Compassion Fatigue?

Children today are plagued by a number of environmental and biological risk factors including family instability, poor nutrition, exposure to toxic chemicals, and abuse. All of these risk factors can lead to negative influences on healthy psychological and physical development. Chapter 2 explores what adverse childhood experiences are and the impact they have on the individual. Trauma affects the developing brain in a variety of ways, and can significantly influence a child's life trajectory. Trauma creates a disruption in a child's normal brain development leaving profound, lasting effects on a child's ability to process information, employ problem/decision-making strategies, and ultimately to learn (Grossman et al., 2003).

There are also possibly negative implications when educators address childhood trauma in the classroom. Trauma not only affects the individual, it also can have a profound effect on the helper. Teachers, school counselors, and administrators can be negatively impacted by the struggles of individual students, as well as suffer from the cumulative burden of supporting all students who have experienced trauma.

This chapter will examine the risk factors that may promote the development of burnout and compassion fatigue among educators. First, we will look at personal attributes associated with greater risk for developing burnout and compassion fatigue. The second part of this chapter will identify the environmental factors that influence the development of burnout and compassion fatigue.

Personal Experience with ACES

The Adverse Childhood Experience Study (ACES) examined the childhood origins that contribute to many of the nation's health and social problems (Anda et al., 2006). The study found that approximately two-thirds of individuals have experienced at least one adverse childhood experience (Anda et al., 2006). The impact that this result has on the current population should not be underestimated, as the number includes many professionals currently working in helping professions, such as counseling and education.

Education professionals encounter a number of risk factors when dealing with trauma in the classroom. The first involves a personal history of an adverse childhood experience. Educators, who themselves may have a history of adverse childhood experiences, are now confronted with children undergoing similar situations.

I mean it just hits you hard. You just don't want to be confrontational and I knew I was coming in with baggage of my own. I didn't know how much of that would affect the [outcome] of the meeting.

(Female teacher, ten years' experience)

ACES exert a profound effect on one's personal development and the way in which they perceive and subsequently handle situations arising with the children in their care. Witnessing the effects of childhood maltreatment has the potential to resurrect an educator's own personal history. In addition, an adult with ACES may experience an impaired ability to cope with daily stressors. If a person does not have the capacity to cope with the demands of daily stressors, chronic stress and anxiety occurs. Individuals who are overworked and emotionally exhausted have less cognitive, emotional, spiritual, and physical energy to manage compassion stress symptoms, leading eventually to the development of burn-out and/or compassion fatigue (Gentry, 2005).

Lack of Training in Trauma

Quality of educator training, including undergraduate training programs, advanced degrees, and opportunities for professional in-service, is an individual risk factor for the development of burnout and compassion fatigue. Years of experience and level of education appears to have little influence on the development of burnout and compassion fatigue when teachers are confronted with trauma-related material.

> *Nobody talks about the emotional toll that it takes when you see these kids in these positions and knowing you can't change it. It keeps you an arm's length away from the emotions of the kids, which is ineffective teaching, or you just keep taking the dings to the point where you just can't do it anymore. I think you lose a lot of good staff that way. I really do. So I think the training would be beneficial, but I think there has to be follow-up. You just can't throw (us) textbook stuff and expect us to absorb it and not give us keys on how to handle the day to day.*

(Female teacher, 27 years' experience)

Preparation programs do little to address childhood trauma in a formal, organized manner, and trauma courses are rarely included or required as a part of the teacher education curriculum. The negative effects of trauma are also the source of a child's difficult adjustment to a classroom environment. Such students exhibiting challenging behaviors can pose problems for teachers, administrators, and paraprofessionals unprepared to effectively handle the situation. Children who are traumatized often have immature, underdeveloped coping mechanisms (Bloom, 1999).

Many educators feel unprepared to deal with the trauma students bring into the school environment. A great number of teachers, school counselors, and administrators developed experience in this area through "natural experiences" occurring in fieldwork or through personal experience. Few educators can identify curriculum that prepared them for dealing with student poverty or childhood trauma.

> *Sometimes I feel that they drop this kid off at your door and "there you go." You learn what's wrong with them and how to deal with it. A lot of times you don't even know what's going on, but you know there is some type of trauma. So I really feel that it is a baptism by fire ... I think training would be, should be greatly improved.*
>
> (Female teacher, ten years' experience)

The very strength that enables teachers to complete their job responsibilities effectively and to have a dramatic impact on the life of a child can also be their undoing. The best teachers are often described as caring, understanding, helpful, and supportive. These traits can create conditions where educators become overwhelmed by the sheer needs of their students. When compassion stress is not addressed effectively, empathy can lead to traumatic stress when teachers are feeling overwhelmed emotionally (Saakvitne & Pearlman, 1996). According to Valent (2002), people can experience feelings of distress and trauma from believing that they have not done enough to avert another individual's suffering. When the individual is a child at high risk, it is suggested that professionals are predisposed to an even greater risk of developing compassion fatigue (Figley, 2002).

Educators often juggle a large number of cases—some involving a Children and Youth Services referral, others are less clear cut—but each case can take the same emotional toll. Often just as much time, energy, concern, and emotion is spent on a child for whom the abuse was only suspected, as for one for whom it was proven. Whether the abuse can actually be proven does not alleviate the impact that child's circumstances will have on the teacher and the classroom.

> *A lot of times, they think that there is nothing wrong, that there is no trauma, and a lot of times they don't really care. It's like they*

think, "They [the teachers] will learn how to deal with them [the traumatized children]."

(Female teacher, ten years' experience)

Unfortunately, accreditation standards across all disciplines of academic human service training programs rarely address the topic of trauma (Levers, 2007). Trauma and poverty are pervasive in today's classroom. If teacher and counselor training programs fail to recognize this matter and address it within their curricula, generations of teachers and school counselors will enter the field inadequately trained and underprepared to address the needs of their students.

The first time I encountered these issues, I was student teaching in a district with a lot of low-income families. I guess during student teaching was the first time I had encountered that ... I hate to say it, but the professors just said, "Well, we'll let the cooperating teachers deal with it." They never really expanded on what to do. Right now, I'm doing my master's program and there is this little blurb of that, like poverty, but it's probably like a paragraph long in the textbook.

(Female teacher, three years' experience)

Lack of professional preparation in this area will continue to perpetuate the cycle of teacher attrition, contributing to a reduction of educators with a more sophisticated level of professional experience who can serve as effective models for newer professionals entering the field. The ultimate goal in having a highly qualified, effective teaching and counseling staff is to provide the maximum educational programming to the children they serve.

There needs to be some follow-up, maybe some kind of coping class. Because I think a lot of good teachers leave the field early because they just can't handle it anymore, and I think what's worse is the ones who can't handle it anymore and stay in the field because they don't know any other job and I see it taking a detrimental toll on kids. They [educators] may have been highly effective for five or ten years, but you can only suffer so many pains of little people and like I said, each one takes a small dent out of you before you start to feel like you either have to put a shield out or love these kids and families. Because if you don't have that connection to them, then you're not going to make the change.

(Female teacher, ten years' experience)

Teacher preparation programs can assist their students by providing the opportunity to discuss hypothetical cases with other professionals who had an expertise in trauma that, in addition to brainstorming various courses of action, would also prove greatly beneficial. Seasoned educators could also instruct on topics such as classroom management, instructional methods, curriculum, and theory, as well as address the practical implications of all of this knowledge. Many supervisors advance up the administrative chain of command because they hold the right credentials and certificate— yet they possess little practical knowledge or formal training that would be helpful to the staff in times of crisis.

Changes in Student Needs

There are a number of societal issues that educators face in the classroom. These include the current state of the economy, an increase in families receiving government aid, children residing in single parent homes, and even homelessness. Poverty can affect children directly and indirectly. A child's health and development can be compromised by poor quality living conditions and limited nutritional options (Pachter, Auinger, Palmer, & Weitzman, 2006).

In a low socio-economic environment, children often lack quality childcare, health care, and educational institutions (Pachter et al., 2006). Family cohesion can be compromised due to lack of employment or consistent, living wages (Pachter et al., 2006). Family instability is further compounded by frequent changes in residence as a result of eviction or moving (Evans, 2004). Impoverished families are also at a 40% higher risk of having a child with an identified disability (Meyers, Lukemeyer, & Smeeding, 1998). Children living in low socio-economic households are also more likely to be exposed to greater levels of abuse and violence (Evans, 2004). As mandated reporters, teachers are often on the front lines confronting issues of abuse and helping the child cope and adjust through the investigative process.

Educators also identify the challenge of changes in student needs, indicating that it seems as if more children in their classrooms are presenting specific, involved global delays than when they first began their careers. One special education teacher noted,

> *I think 10 years ago, I had maybe one child who was autistic, two children with Down syndrome, and the rest were speech impaired. Now, most of my kids are on the autism spectrum or more profoundly delayed.*
>
> (Male teacher, ten years' experience)

With the goal of providing an inclusive environment for all students, educators are working with a wider range of social, developmental, and physical issues. Educators interact often with the families of their students and are asked to wear many hats. Depending on the type of childhood trauma a student faces, educators are asked to play the role of teacher, counselor, social worker, and administrator on a daily basis.

Quality of Professional Support

Another environmental factor that influences the development of burnout and compassion fatigue is the quality of available professional support for educators. Administrative support is a determinant of teacher self-efficacy and job satisfaction. It appears consistently in teacher attrition research literature as a mitigating factor to teacher success.

> *I think it's extremely important. You have to have a strong admin-istrative team to even be able to support the teacher to get through. I know that with my supervisor, there have been days where I have called her, burned out, saying, "They say they hate me." Just look-ing for the reassurance that "Yeah, I'm a good teacher." I have always thought that. I think it is very important.*
>
> (Female teacher, nine years' experience)

The important role that an administrator plays in a teacher's professional life has profound effects on the teacher's percep-tion of self-efficacy and compassion satisfaction.

> *I think if we didn't have our administration supporting us, we would have really struggled a lot. It would have been difficult to get through that situation ... I was very thankful that they were there and they supported and believed what was occurring.*
>
> (Male teacher, ten years' experience)

Educators often describe two common types of supervisor sup-port. The Involved Supervisor provides clear expectations, un-equivocal support, constructive feedback, validation of teacher efforts, and most important, emotional support.

> *There was never really an issue where I was calling my supervisor and going, "Now where do I put this or where do I put that?" Mine was always more, "I had a really bad day and this kid did this and I need some help." So that was more important to me than the other stuff.*
>
> (Female teacher, nine years' experience)

A Detached Supervisor is far removed from the day-today class-room activities, provides little follow through on important mat-ters, is more involved in administrative tasks, emotionally and professionally unavailable, and provides little to no support. A Detached Supervisor creates conditions that promote the devel-opment of burnout and compassion fatigue.

I think [administrative support] is extremely important. I think administrative support with anything is probably the most important thing. When you don't have an administrator that supports you or even understands the situation … they are not going to have much sympathy.

(Female teacher, ten years' experience)

Administrative support is important when addressing student trauma. In these cases, the supervisor should acknowledge the veracity of the information presented about the child.

I think it's very important that administrators acknowledge that this [trauma] is present and provide support, or resources, or staff.

(Female teacher, ten years' experience)

Consulting administration can sometimes be seen as the last step in trying to handle an incident of child maltreatment. Even though educators often agree upon the importance of having an effective administrator, some also report that they only accessed administration when absolutely necessary. In their words, administration was called for "big things."

Sometimes I think you're afraid to tell your administrator something because they are going to think you don't know how to teach or you don't know how to deal with the situation yourself.

(Female teacher, ten years' experience)

Sometimes, it is challenging to work with administration when they don't sense an administrator is going to provide the necessary support.

We can utilize a supervisor, but a lot of times it's just easier to deal in house. I think just because we are the ones seeing them [the children] every day. It's hard to get an outside perspective when they don't know the kids or what is going on.

(Female teacher, ten years' experience)

An experience of having a detached supervisor is as follows:

I don't have that support from our main administrator. I don't know if it's because we have been there so long that she almost feels like we can run it ourselves. And there are times when we really do need that person to help us and we don't get the help... [When handling a child abuse issue] our administrator really wasn't involved. Asked a few questions once in a while, but nothing too much.
(Female teacher, 12 years' experience)

Billingsley and Cross (1992) determined that regular and special educators felt more social connectedness, a higher degree of responsibility to their jobs, and a lower level of stress when they received administrative support. Support from other educators can be crucial in lowering stress levels and improving job satisfaction. Often, collegial support from para-professional staff, instead of other teachers, can be essential in helping to de-brief from stressful and traumatic situations.

If I didn't have another person in that room, I think it would be difficult to continue on some days without having a person there to talk to about stressful situations immediately ... So, just having the folks that I work with on a day-to-day basis there to talk is a good resource.
(Male teacher, ten years' experience)

Caseloads

Environmental factors such as long work hours and high caseloads have also been associated with increased risk of burnout and compassion fatigue (Boscarino, Figley, & Adams, 2004; Creamer & Liddle, 2005; Meyers & Cornille, 2002). However, the number of students is only one aspect of an educator's caseload. Caseload quantity should also be measured according to frequency of interaction with students. How often do you see the students in your caseload? Once a week? Daily? Another measure of quantity is duration. For how long do you interact with your students? Are they in your classroom all day? Fifty minutes?

Another important issue to consider when examining educator caseloads is not only the quantity, but also the quality of the caseload. Interpersonal distance is one aspect of an educator's caseload. How closely do you typically interact with your students? In large group settings? One-on-one? In the case of special education teachers, they may find themselves providing not only cognitive and emotional intimacy, but physical intimacy as well. A special education teacher's caseload could also include caring for students' physical needs, such as wiping noses, assisting them dress, toileting, etc.

The impact of one's caseload should also be measured by characteristics of the students, such as their ages and particular needs. You may find yourself shouldering a larger emotional burden for younger students who are developmentally unable to understand or adequately cope with traumatic experiences. Also, the depth of trauma your students are dealing with affects your risk levels as well. Educators with high caseloads of children who have survived violent or human-induced trauma appear to be at greater risk for burnout and compassion fatigue (Creamer & Liddle, 2005; Cunningham, 2003).

It is important to remember that students who have experienced trauma suffer from severe symptoms that can significantly affect the educators who work with them over the long haul. Whenever possible, a best practice would be to develop an optimal "caseload mix" that balances the various needs of students among the staff in a building. Purposely structuring classrooms with students presenting with easier problems can help to mitigate the effects of working with students who present with more difficult, and in some cases, intractable, problems (Jackson, Schwab, & Schuler, 1986).

Additional Resources

The following is a link to the Adverse Childhood Experiences quiz. This article also provides resources for learning more about the ACES survey and what your score may mean in terms of your own overall physical and mental health. https://www. npr.org/sections/health-shots/2015/03/02/387007941/ take-the-ace-quiz-and-learn-what-it-does-and-doesnt-mean

Nakazawa, D. J. (2015). *Childhood disrupted: How your biography becomes your biology, and how you can heal.* New York, NY: Simon and Schuster.

Payne, R. K., DeVol, P., & Smith, T. D. (2009). *Bridges out of poverty: Strategies for professionals and communities.* New York, NY: Aha! Process, Inc.

The following are free resources to support you in your efforts to mitigate the effects of poverty in creating high achieving, healthy school communities: https://www. ahaprocess.com/solutions/k-12-schools/events-resources/ free-resources/

Self-Reflective Questions for Thoughtful Practice

Each educator carries their own unique set of risk factors for developing burnout and compassion fatigue. This chapter discussed a number of risk factors for you to reflect on in terms of your own personal characteristics and your work environment. Answer the questions thoughtfully below as you begin to assess your own risk levels.

In the "Additional Resources" section of this chapter, there is a link to an Adverse Childhood Experiences survey. What is your ACES score? How might that score influence your risk for burnout and compassion fatigue?

_____

_____

_____

_____

How would you describe the availability of administrative support in your work environment? How might this influence your risk for burnout and compassion fatigue?

_____

_____

_____

_____

How would you describe your current caseload of students? How does the quantity and quality of their needs contribute to your feelings of stress?

_____

_____

_____

_____

References

Anda, R. F., Felitti, V. J., Walker, J., Whitfield, C. L., Cremner, J. D., Perry, B. D., Dube, S. R., & Giles, W. H. (2006). The enduring effects of abuse and related adverse experiences in childhood: A convergence of evidence from the neurobiology and epidemiology. *European Archives of Psychiatry & Clinical Neurosciences, 256*(3), 174–186.

Billingsley, B. S., & Cross, L. H. (1992). Predictors of commitment, job satisfaction, and intent to stay in teaching: A comparison of general and special educators. *The Journal of Special Education, 25*(4), 453–471.

Bloom S. L. (1999). Trauma theory abbreviated. *Final action plan: A coordinated community-based response to family violence.* Retrieved on December 10, 2018 from http://www.sanctuaryweb.com/Documents/Trauma%20theory%20abbreviated.pdf

Boscarino, J. A., Figley, C. R., & Adams, R. E. (2004). Compassion fatigue following the September 11 terrorist attacks: A study of secondary trauma among New York City social workers. *International Journal of Emergency Mental Health, 6*(2), 57.

Creamer, T. L., & Liddle, B. J. (2005). Secondary traumatic stress among disaster mental health workers responding to the September 11 attacks. *Journal of Traumatic Stress: Official Publication of the International Society for Traumatic Stress Studies, 18*(1), 89–96.

Cunningham, M. (2003). Impact of trauma work on social work clinicians: Empirical findings. *Social Work, 48*(4), 451–459.

Evans, G. (2004). The environment of childhood poverty. *The American Psychologist, 59*(2), 77–92.

Figley, C. R. (Ed.). (2002). *Treating compassion fatigue* (1st ed.). New York, NY: Brunner-Routledge.

Gentry, J. E. (2005). *Compassion fatigue: Prevention and resiliency.* Eau Claire, WI: PESI Healthcare, LLC.

Grossman, A. W., Churchill, J. D., McKinney, B. C., Kodish, I. M., Otte, S. L., & Greenough, W. T. (2003). Experience effects on brain development: Possible contributions to psychopathology. *Journal of Child Psychology and Psychiatry, 44*(1), 33–63.

Jackson, S. E., Schwab, R. L., & Schuler, R. S. (1986). Toward an understanding of the burnout phenomenon. *Journal of Applied Psychology, 71*(4), 630.

Levers, L. L. (2007). On being a professional counselor. In J. Gregoire & C. M. Jungers (Eds.), *The Counselor's Companion.* London, England: Lawrence Erlbaum Associates.

Meyers, M., Lukemeyer, A., & Smeeding, T. (1998). The cost of caring: Childhood disability and poor families. *Social Service Review, 72,* 209–234.

Meyers, T. W., & Cornille, T. (2002). The trauma of working with traumatized children. In C. R. Figley (Ed.), *Treating compassion fatigue* (39–55). New York, NY: Brunner-Routledge.

Pachter, L. M., Auinger, P., Palmer, R., Weitzman, M. (2006). Do parenting and the home environment, maternal depression, neighborhood, and chronic poverty affect child behavioral problems differently in different racial-ethnic groups? *Pediatrics, 117*(4), 1329–1338.

Saakvitne, K. W. & Pearlman, L. A. (1996). *Transforming the pain: A workbook on vicarious traumatization.* New York: W. W. Norton & Company.

Valent, P. (2002). Diagnosis and treatment of helper stresses, trauma, and illnesses. In C. R. Figley (Ed.), *Treating compassion fatigue* (1st ed., pp. 17–38). New York, NY: Brunner-Routledge.

4

BURNOUT
Death by a Thousand Cuts

Things That Make You Go *Hmmm*

A growing body of research demonstrates that the topic of burn-out among teachers is gaining traction in the United States and abroad. Consider the following facts:

- About half a million (15%) of teachers leave the profession every year (Seidel, 2014).
- More than 41% of teachers leave the profession within five years of starting, and teacher attrition has risen significantly over the last two decades (Ingersoll, Merrill, and Stuckey, 2014).
- Almost 66% of the nation's best teachers continue to leave the profession for careers elsewhere (Chartock & Wiener, 2014).

While the percentage of teachers who leave the field due to burnout are unclear, we do have a better understanding about what influences the development of burnout in educators. Some of the factors that contribute to educator burnout are listed below. Do any of these pertain to you?

- High caseload numbers, lack of professional experience, role identification/ambiguity (Cross & Billingsley, 1994; Gersten et al., 2001);
- Lack of resources (Edmonson & Thompson, 2002);
- Lack of administrative support (Billingsley, 2004);

- Inadequate salary (Singer, 1993);
- Negative school climate and insufficient colleague support (Miller et al., 1999);
- Increased paperwork (Billingsley et al., 1995; Gersten et al., 2001) and;
- High levels of stress (Gersten et al., 2001; Singh & Billingsley, 1996).

What is Burnout?

Unfortunately, there is little agreement among many research-ers as to what burnout is and what causes it. This lack of under-standing is one of the reasons burnout can be a difficult issue to address. The American psychologist Herbert Freudenberger (1974) coined the term *burnout* to describe the consequences of severe stress in the helping professions. Freudenberger de-scribed burnout as a "feeling of exhaustion and fatigue" (p. 160). Another researcher, Christina Maslach (2015), describes burn-out as "a response to the chronic emotional strain of dealing extensively with other human beings, particularly when they are troubled or having problems" (p. 2).

Maslach and Jackson (1981) defined burnout as "a syndrome of emotional exhaustion and cynicism that occurs in individuals who do 'people work' of some kind" (p. 99). Teaching is cer-tainly people work! On any given day, you have the potential to interact with students, fellow teachers, parents, administration, and/or members of the local community. In addition, the peo-ple you most closely work with could be ages five, 12, or 17 which certainly adds another challenging dimension!

Sources of Burnout

What leads to an educator developing burnout? Burnout in the workplace is often the result of a mismatch between the per-son and the work environment. However, according to Maslach (2015), there are three specific sources that influence the devel-opment of burnout. The first source involves the dynamics of the interactions one has with a variety of individuals in the school setting. The second source of burnout is situated within the work environment that those interactions take place. Last, it is important to explore the individual characteristics that may influence one's likelihood of developing burnout.

Dynamics of Interactions

"People work" can be very demanding! As an educator, it takes a lot of energy to interact with people all day—to remain calm when faced with challenges, patient when frustrated, and understanding when met by an unending list of student needs. Involvement with people is one source of burnout. Specifically, the nature of an educator's involvement with others influences the development of burnout.

A common characteristic among those experiencing burnout is a shift in one's view of other people. When burnout occurs, you begin to develop a negative and uncaring approach towards others. This negative approach is influenced by an approach to students that focuses mainly on their weaknesses, deficiencies, and problems. In addition, teachers often don't get positive feedback when students are succeeding and things are going well. Lopsided relationships with administrators, community, or students themselves can make the whole teaching experience seem rather unrewarding.

When the nature of an educator's contact with students is especially upsetting, depressing, or difficult, it can exacerbate the levels of emotional stress one experiences. For example, teachers working with students from high poverty environments may feel helpless to respond to their students' needs, to change their students' circumstances, or to cure larger societal problems. Sometimes the development of burnout can also be influenced by the likability of others. We often think about the students we teach as either "good" students or "bad" students. Those who fall into the "bad" category may be demanding of our attention, resistant to learning, and unmanageable behaviorally. These students require more of our effort, and often make our time with them seem unpleasant.

Lastly, how you relate to others in the educational setting influences the development of burnout. When students struggle with issues that have personal relevance to you, it can affect you by bringing up unpleasant memories or unresolved feelings. A natural response may be to empathize with your students. However, taking on students' feelings as your own creates an enormous emotional load that can quickly lead to exhaustion and burnout. The same is true when teachers get too highly involved with students on a personal level. A lack of clear boundaries can enable you to become too emotionally involved with your students' problems and needs.

Workplace Environment

There are seven domains of the workplace environment that contribute to burnout (Leiter & Maslach, 2008). The first is associated with *workload*. Work overload is an everyday occurrence in the life of an educator. Work overload can stem from:

- Confusion over roles and responsibilities (Billingsley et al., 1995; Cross & Billingsley, 1994; Singh & Billingsley, 1996);
- Management of the increasing volume of paperwork (Westling & Whitten, 1996);
- Changes in service delivery models (Morvant et al., 1995) and;
- Increasing student caseloads (Morvant et al., 1995).

Teaching is a field that requires full days in the classroom and many hours beyond that to lesson plan, grade assignments, and complete paperwork. Teachers also spend time working one-on-one with students, meeting with other teaching staff and administrators, and communicating with parents. On average, teachers report working 53 hours per week (Scholastic, Inc. and Bill & Melinda Gates Foundation, 2014).

A second source of burnout in the workplace environment is a *lack of control* over classroom, school, and district policies.

Teachers have little or no control over much of the decision-making that affects their role and lack the ability to change many of the factors that contribute to teacher stress and burnout. People in high performance jobs can cope if they have support and autonomy. However, teachers often experience the opposite. Managing new curriculum changes and new initiatives while demonstrating student improvement in learning with limited resources and support creates high levels of stress among educators.

Insufficient reward is the third source of environmental burnout among educators. Most educators do not enter the field for monetary rewards. However, low salaries do impact a teacher's susceptibility to burnout, especially if a teacher salary makes it difficult to achieve middle-class milestones, such as paying off student loans, purchasing a house, or sending a child to college. Other rewards come in the form of a teacher's perception of positive recognition. When such support is absent, lack of reward becomes a contributing factor to burnout (Leiter & Maslach, 1999).

Another component that Leiter and Maslach (1999) identified as contributing to the overall concept of burnout is an individual's perception of administrative and organizational *fairness*. Decisions about work assignments, schedules, and rewards should be consistent, predictable, and transparent. When educators believe that they are respected and valued, they are more likely to feel a sense of community with their colleagues and to develop a sense of trust within the organization.

Breakdown of community is the fifth source of environmental educator burnout. Miller et al. (1999) found that collegial support has strong associations with determining if a teacher will stay in education or leave. Teachers are four times more likely to stay in their current positions if they perceive administrative leadership as supportive (Boe et al., 2008). Administrative and collegial support, which engenders a climate of professional rewards and recognition, can contribute significantly to the creation of a safe, positive working environment that wards off burnout.

Finally, burnout is likely to occur when individuals experience a conflict between personal and organization *values* (Leiter & Maslach, 1999). Educators may feel that they are being asked to do meaningless work or to do their work in ways that are wrong or unethical. An example might be the struggle educators feel about wanting to teach in ways that are best for students when policies limit those opportunities due to the pressure of performance testing (Santoro, 2011). This sense of demoralization can produce feelings of helplessness and discouragement, which in turn may lead to burnout.

Individual Qualities

Individual qualities and characteristics also determine how someone handles stress, which help to explain why one person may develop burnout while another person may not. An examination of internal factors can help us determine who is more at risk for burnout. Table 4.1 provides an overview of demographic and personality characteristics that influence the development of burnout.

Table 4.1 **Personal Characteristics as a Source of Burnout**

Demographic Characteristics	
Sex	Overall, men and women tend to experience burnout at similar rates. Women tend to experience emotional exhaustion, while men are more likely to have depersonalized and negative feelings about the people they work with.
Race	Black helping professionals tend not to burn out at as high rates as white helping professionals.
Age	Burnout occurs more frequently in young professionals
Marital and Family Status	Single workers experience the most burnout, while married workers experience it the least. Workers with children tend to be less vulnerable to burnout.
Education	Burnout is highest among those with bachelor's degrees but no postgraduate education.

Personality Characteristics

Self-Concept	Those who lack self-esteem and confidence are more vulnerable to burnout. Failure to set and recognize personal limits also contributes to burnout.
Personal Needs	The need to be liked and approved of is strongly related to the development of burnout. A high need to achieve and an excessive need for control also contributes to the development of burnout.
Personal Motivations	Those who see themselves as "rescuers", or seek intimacy and affection through the helping relationship are more prone to burnout.
Emotional Control	Individuals who struggle to appropriately express anger or cope with fear are more likely to develop burnout. The inability to empathize with someone without vicariously living their experience will significantly contribute to the development of burnout.

Maslach (2015)

"I. Just. Can't. Even." and Other Signs of Burnout

The term burnout is often inaccurately used to casually describe a bad day or a bad week. However, burnout is not a temporary condition. For someone truly experiencing burnout, it is a chronic state of feeling overworked, overwhelmed, and exhausted. The symptoms of burnout affect one's mental, emotional, and physical states. What follows is a comprehensive list of the symptoms of burnout (Carter, 2012). Knowing the signs and symptoms of burnout can help you identify it and reverse the downward spiral.

Maslach and Jackson (1981) described burnout as "a syndrome of emotional exhaustion and cynicism that occurs in individuals who do 'people work' of some kind" (p. 99). They identified the three dimensions of burnout as being:

- An overwhelming exhaustion;
- Feelings of cynicism and detachment from the job and;
- A sense of ineffectiveness and lack of accomplishment.

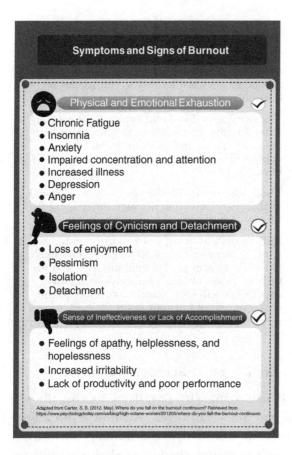

Figure 4.1 **Symptoms and signs of burnout.**

Exhaustion refers to feelings of being overextended as well as the depletion of emotional and physical resources (Maslach, Shaufeli, & Leiter, 2001). When an individual suffers from burnout, extreme emotional and physical exhaustion is experienced. Exhaustion is often the first sign that the stressors of one's job have become too demanding (Leiter & Maslach, 1999). The following are some symptoms of physical and emotional exhaustion:

•   *Chronic fatigue.* Low energy and often feeling tired are common symptoms of early stages of burnout. You might go to bed early, but still wake up tired. Or you might lack energy and motivation to tackle daily routine tasks. In later stages of burnout, you may feel drained, and completely lacking in energy. Some people may find it difficult to get out of bed. Emotionally, it may manifest as a sense of dread about the coming day.

- *Insomnia.* Individuals in the early stages of burnout might experience sleep difficulties a few nights a week. Sleep difficulties may include the inability to fall asleep, stay asleep, or waking up too early. You may find that your inability to sleep is directly affected by persistent thoughts about your workload and the challenge of getting everything done. In later stages of burnout, insomnia can become a nightly occurrence, perhaps even reaching the point where you may not be able to sleep at all some nights.

- *Impaired concentration.* Lack of concentration, attention difficulties, and forgetfulness are common cognitive problems associated with burnout. You might find yourself unable to remember details, or you might struggle to focus on what you are reading or hearing. Your inability to focus can create more stress as it takes longer to get your work done. In late stages of burnout, these symptoms may prevent you from getting anything accomplished.

- *Increased illness.* Chronic stress negatively impacts a person's immune system. Therefore, victims of burnout are susceptible to colds, flu, and other illnesses. The worse the burnout is, the more vulnerable you are to illnesses, and it will likely take you longer to recover.

- *Loss of appetite.* In the early stages of burnout, loss of appetite might affect your ability to feel hunger. You may find yourself missing meals, or not eating nourishing, balanced meals. In later stages, you may suffer a complete loss of appetite which could result in significant, unhealthy weight loss.

- *Anxiety.* Feelings of tension, worry, and edginess may affect your ability to pay attention and concentrate in early stages of burnout. This may develop into chronic anxiety, and over time, could interfere with your ability to go to work or manage responsibilities in your personal life. The anxiety may become so severe that you experience panic attacks.

- *Depression.* During the early stages of burnout, you may notice that you are having more bad days than good days. Some experience their depression as a general unhappiness and loss of confidence. It is also common to experience feelings of guilt and worthlessness. As depression worsens, individuals may experience distorted thinking, where everything seems bleak. Individuals may hold extremely negative views about themselves, their situation, and the future. Feeling hopeless and helpless, individuals may even think about suicide.
- *Anger.* Victims of burnout often feel as if they failed, and experience guilt because of it. These feelings may turn into anger and resentment. This anger might be the source of interpersonal tension with students, colleagues, and personal relationships. As burnout becomes more severe, that anger may intensify and result in angry outbursts and serious arguments. At its most extreme, this anger could take a violent turn.

In an effort to cope with increasing levels of physical and emotional exhaustion, teachers may distance themselves from their students or begin to develop negative attitudes or feelings toward their students (Jennett, Harris, & Mesibov, 2003). This sense of depersonalization leads to the second dimension of burnout, which includes indifference and adoption of a cynical attitude toward the work. Depersonalization entails a negative or excessively detached response to a variety of experiences within the job role. The following are symptoms associated with depersonalization:

- *Loss of enjoyment.* In the beginning stages of burnout, you may feel a loss of enjoyment about your role as an educator. You don't enjoy going to work, and when you get there, you can't wait to leave. As burnout intensifies, you may experience a loss of enjoyment in other areas of your life, including time spent with family and friends. At work, you may seek to avoid projects or become preoccupied with how you might escape work responsibilities entirely.

- *Pessimism.* Burnout can affect how you see the world. Before becoming burned out, you may have approached your work with enthusiasm and optimism. Now you might approach your work with a negative outlook, such as the expectation that nothing is going to turn out well. This negative perspective may also be directed at others, where you might feel that no one cares or that everyone is out for themselves. A lack of trust towards others might promote tension in your relationships with others and prevent you from engaging in the social support that once may have assisted you in handling stress.

- *Isolation.* This may start out as mild resistance, such as avoiding socializing with co-workers or friends. With increasing levels of burnout, your desire to be alone intensifies. Co-workers stopping by to chat may become an annoyance, and you might find excuses to keep your classroom door or office door shut. You may also find excuses to get out of meetings, and find yourself changing behavior patterns to avoid interaction with others. You may even get angry when you are approached by others.

- *Detachment.* When dealing with burnout, detachment is characterized by a feeling of disconnection from people and your environment. This can occur by engaging in isolating behaviors, or may manifest itself as anger towards others. When you detach yourself emotionally and physically from your job and other responsibilities, it may be in the form of calling in sick more often, missing appointments, being chronically late, or not returning phone calls, emails, or texts.

The next sign of burnout, reduced personal accomplishment, refers to "feelings of incompetence and a lack of achievement and productivity at work" (Maslach, 2015, p. 7). In this dimension of burnout, educators have an increasing sense of inadequacy about their ability to respond to and educate students.

This may influence a growing sense of failure. The following are symptoms associated with a sense of ineffectiveness and lack of accomplishment:

- *Apathy.* With apathy comes the feelings of helplessness and hopelessness. In the beginning stages of burnout, educators may feel as if nothing is going right, or there really isn't any point in putting forth so much effort. These feelings may become immobilizing, making it difficult to see the worth in doing anything at all. With extreme cases of burnout, educators may not see why they should bother showing up for work, or even get out of bed.
- *Increased irritability.* With burnout, irritability often stems from frustration over feeling unsuccessful and ineffective. Teachers may feel disappointment over their lack of productivity, and lowered quality of their work performance. You may speak sharply with people and overreact to minor things. Irritability might negatively affect your personal and professional relationships. In later stages of burnout, it may manifest itself in arguments, broken and strained relationships, and even divorce.
- *Lack of productivity/poor performance.* The most visible impact of burnout is the change in one's work performance. With impaired outlook comes a change in your approach to your work. There may not be as much care or creativity in developing lesson plans, or concern about students achieving learning outcomes. Rather than doing work badly, you may simply do less of it. You might avoid all unnecessary tasks ("That's not my job/responsibility") and limit the length of instruction or time spent working individually with students.

How Do I Know if I am Experiencing Burnout?

It can be helpful to think about burnout as a series of stages through which the effects of burnout increase in intensity. Veninga and Spradley's (1981) model describes five stages that can assist educators in assessing their risk of burnout.

Stage One is the *honeymoon* stage, characterized by high job satisfaction, commitment, energy, and creativity. Educators are highly engaged. In this stage, the patterns of coping with job stress are important in determining the trajectory of risk for burnout. Individuals who are able to develop positive and adaptive resiliency strategies will be able to maintain higher levels of job engagement and satisfaction.

Stage Two is known as *fuel shortage*, in which the reality of the daily life of the job begins to set in. This stage is marked by periods of job dissatisfaction and work inefficiency. Individuals may find themselves procrastinating and struggling to keep track of details associated with their professional roles. Sometimes educators may experience fatigue that can be exacerbated by the inability to fall asleep at night. Some report that thinking about work issues made it difficult to "shut their brain down." Negative ways of coping with job stress begin to take hold, such as overeating, drinking, and smoking as well as escapist activities such as excessive napping, binge-watching TV, or playing video games. Burnout at this stage is more easily addressed if immediate intervention occurs.

Stage Three is characterized by *chronic symptoms.* This stage is marked by an intensification of the symptoms discussed in Stage Two. Educators experience chronic exhaustion, physical illness, anger, and depression. These symptoms are intense, pervasive, and long-lasting. At this stage, you may find yourself disengaging from the job. Educators can become increasingly prone to illness as the psychological strain manifests itself in physical ways. This may require frequent or ongoing absences from work. The individual attitude towards work continues to decline, and interactions with students, parents, co-workers, friends, and family members undergo a noticeable negative shift.

Stage Four is the *crisis* stage. In this stage, the symptoms become critical. Physical symptoms of stress intensify or increase in number. Educators may begin to obsess about their work frustrations, coloring all aspects of their life. Pessimism and self-doubt dominate thoughts, and the individual develops an "escapist mentality." However, withdrawal from or avoidance of work responsibilities can result in plummeting productivity and negative assessment of work performance. Withdrawal can also damage personal and professional relationships and further isolate one from supportive social circles.

Stage Five is what is often called *hitting the wall* and is characterized by professional incompetence and total impairment. In this stage, the symptoms of burnout are so embedded in an individual's life that it can be labeled as a significant physical or emotional problem. If burnout is not identified early and mitigated, it can lead to very serious issues for student educators. Those who are experiencing some levels of burnout and then are subsequently exposed to student trauma are more likely to develop compassion fatigue.

Another way to assess whether you suffer from burnout is using the *Professional Quality of Life Scale* (ProQOL) located in Appendix B at the back of this book. The ProQOL measures negative and positive aspects of being a helper using three sub-scales: burnout, compassion satisfaction, and compassion fatigue. A high score on the burnout sub-section of the ProQOL means that you are at higher risk for developing burnout.

What Can Be Done to Combat Burnout?

Burnout is both a personal and organizational problem. However, burnout tends to be framed as a problem with the person, and solutions overwhelmingly focus on addressing perceived individual inadequacies in dealing with stress. Most approaches to burnout are preventative, such as developing resiliency skills to assist you in coping with, or better managing workplace stressors. Other approaches focus on those in the latter stages of burnout, with the goal of reducing the unhealthy deficits acquired under pervasive and chronic stress. Chapter 7 in this book will provide detailed approaches to increase individual resiliency and prevent burnout.

Additional Resources

Rankin, J. (2017). *First aid for teacher burnout.* New York: Routledge.

The following is a link to the Teaching Tolerance Fall 2015 newsletter that focuses on educator burnout. On page 2 is a self-scoring quiz to assess if you are experiencing burnout.

http://www.tolerance.org/sites/default/files/general/Teaching%20Tolerance%2051%20ED%20Cafe.pdf

Sponsored by the *How I Decide Foundation,* this link will take you to a series of seven short videos called "Burnout Blockers" that apply habit psychology and decision science to promote resiliency among teachers.

https://www.youtube.com/channel/UC5qYkn8DdYPO GW24PvHa_dQ/videos

Self-Reflective Questions for Thoughtful Practice

Burnout is a condition that can be brought on by qualities associated with the individual, as well as qualities associated with the work environment. The questions below will allow you to begin to examine the ways in which you may be experiencing burnout. Please take a moment to reflect on factors that may make you vulnerable to burnout.

What experiences do you have at work that could contribute to the development of burnout?

_____

_____

_____

_____

Review the list of the signs and symptoms of burnout. Have you experienced any of these? To what degree?

_____

_____

_____

_____

What individual qualities (Table 4.1) do you possess that might make you vulnerable to the development of burnout?

_____

_____

_____

_____

References

Billingsley, B. S. (2004). Special education teacher retention and attrition: A critical analysis of the literature. *Center on Personnel Studies in Special Education, RS-2,* 1–47.

Billingsley, B., Pyecha, J., Smith-Davis, J., Murray, K., & Hendricks, M. B. (1995). *Improving the retention of special education teachers: Final report.* Research Triangle Institute (Prepared for Office of Special Education Programs, Office of Special Education and Rehabilitative Services, US Department of Education under Cooperative Agreement 11023Q10001).(ERIC Document Reproduction Service No. ED379860).

Boe, E. E., Cook, L. H., & Sunderland, R. J. (2008). Teacher turnover: Examining exit attrition, teaching area transfer, and school migration. *Exceptional Children, 75*(1), 7–31.

Carter, S. B. (2012, May). *Where do you fall on the burnout continuum?* Retrieved from https://www.psychologytoday.com/us/blog/high-octane-women/201205/where-do-you-fall-the-burnout-continuum

Chartock, J., & Wiener, R. (2014, November 13). How to save teachers from burning out, dropping out and other hazards of experience. *The Hechinger Report.* Retrieved from http://hechingerreport.org/content/can-keep-great-teachers-engaged-effective-settle-careers_18026

Cross, L. H., & Billingsley, B. S. (1994). Testing a model of special educators' intent to stay in teaching. *Exceptional Children, 60*(5), 411–421.

Edmonson, S., & Thompson, D. (2002). Burnout among special educators. *Toward Wellness: Prevention, Coping, and Stress,* 159–190.

Freudenberger, H. (1974) Staff burnout. *Journal of Social Issues, 30,* 159–165. http://dx.doi.org/10.1111/j.1540-4560.1974.tb00706.x

Gersten, R., Keating, T., Yovanoff, P., & Harniss, M. K. (2001). Working in special education: Factors that enhance special educators' intent to stay. *Exceptional Children, 67*(4), 549–567.

Ingersoll, R.; Merrill, L. & Stuckey, D. (2014). Seven trends: The transformation of the teaching force. *CPRE Research Reports.* Retrieved from https://repository.upenn.edu/cpre_researchreports/79

Jennett, H. K., Harris, S. L., & Mesibov, G. B. (2003). Commitment to philosophy, teacher efficacy, and burnout among teachers of children with autism. *Journal of Autism and Developmental Disorders, 33*(6), 583–593.

Leiter, M. P., & Maslach, C. (1999). Six areas of worklife: A model of the organizational context of burnout. *Journal of Health and Human Services Administration,* 472–489.

Leiter, M. P., & Maslach, C. (2008). Early predictors of job burnout and engagement. *Journal of Applied Psychology, 93*(3), 498–512.

Maslach, C. (2015). *Burnout: The cost of caring.* Los Altos, CA: Malor Books.

Maslach, C., & Jackson, S. E. (1981). The measurement of experienced burnout. *Journal of Occupational Behavior, 2,* 99–113.

Maslach, C., Schaufeli, W. B., & Leiter, M. P. (2001). Job burnout. *Annual Review of Psychology, 52,* 397–422.

Miller, M. D., Brownell, M. T., & Smith, S. W. (1999). Factors that predict teachers staying in, leaving, or transferring from the special education classroom. *Exceptional Children, 65*(2), 201–218.

Morvant, M., Gersten, R., Gillman, J., Keating, T., & Blake, G. (1995). *Attrition/ retention of urban special education teachers: Multi-faceted research and strategic action planning.* Final performance report, Vol. 1. (ERIC Document Reproduction Service No. ED 338 154)

Santoro, D. A. (2011). Good teaching in difficult times: Demoralization in the pursuit of good work. *American Journal of Education, 118*(1), 1–23.

Scholastic, Inc. and Bill & Melinda Gates Foundation. (2014). *Primary sources: America's Teachers on teaching in an era of change,* Third Edition. New York, NY. (ERIC Document Reproduction Service No. ED 562664)

Seidel, A. (2014). The teacher dropout crisis. *National Public Radio.* Retrieved from https://www.npr.org/sections/ed/2014/07/18/332343240/the-teacher-dropout-crisis

Singer, J. D. (1993). Are special educators' career paths special? Results from a 13-year longitudinal study. *Exceptional Children, 59*(3), 262–279.

Singh, K., & Billingsley, B. S. (1996). Intent to stay in teaching: Teachers of students with emotional disorders versus other special educators. *Remedial and Special Education, 17*(1), 37–47.

Westling, D. L., & Whitten, T. M. (1996). Rural special education teachers' plans to continue or leave their teaching positions. *Exceptional Children, 62*(4), 319–335.

Veninga, R. L., & Spradley, J. P. (1981). The *work stress connection: How to cope with job burnout.* Boston, MA: Little, Brown and Company.

5

COMPASSION FATIGUE
Sick, Tired, and Depleted

I noticed an increased heart rate. I had a difficult time expressing what needed to be done. I was a lot more on edge. I just shut down at home. I had a hard time functioning with my [own] children, my spouse. The first week and a half, it took me a good three hours to fall asleep."

(Male special education teacher, 10 years' experience)

Sadly, a paucity of literature exists in the field of education examining compassion fatigue as it relates to secondary trauma. Catastrophic events such as 9/11, devastating weather phenomena such as Hurricanes Katrina and Harvey, and school shootings such as Columbine have been the primary focus of researchers examining this occurrence in K-12 education (Jaycox et al., 2007; Lantieri & Nambiar, 2004). Educators must carry a professional load that is inherently stressful. You are interfacing daily with children who may be experiencing chronic difficulties such as poverty and/or disabilities. On any given day, you are a teacher, counselor, nurse, nose-wiper, and somedays—all-around problem-solver.

Anyone working with at-risk children holds onto that one memory of the child that will haunt them until the end of their days. For me, it is the haunted, disconnected look of a three-year-old shell of a girl who was being sexually abused by her older brothers and the countless stream of men that Mom was allowing into the house. Even though I met her 15 years ago, I can still create a clear image in my mind of her beautiful but vacant eyes.

Educators working with high-needs populations have additional stressors inherent with this particular group. As a result of these ongoing interactions, your exposure to your students' trauma and/or suffering occurs regularly. Kanter (2007) asserts that the degree to which these interactions affect the helper—in this case, educators—are based on the helper's perception of the suffering. All of the things that connect human beings to one another gradually erode when a person is experiencing compassion fatigue. The appearance of compassion fatigue can take many shapes: a diminishing sense of hope, compassion, and empathy; changes in work performance; feelings of bitterness towards our jobs; violation of boundaries; and a loss of emotional regulation. Compassion fatigue does not discriminate—it can affect anyone in a caregiving role. Coincidentally, stressed and traumatized professionals tend to work longer hours and more rigorously, which can exacerbate the problem if not effectively addressed (Mathieu, 2012). As it takes hold, we become increasingly less able to see its daily impact.

Educators wear a variety of hats. Empathy and compassion, critical in helping professions, are employed frequently in teaching. Empathy, often viewed as a psychological strength, can also serve as a potential risk factor for educators who go on to develop compassion stress and fatigue. Care, empathy, devotion, responsibility, nurture, and preservation—all critical psychological and social components of compassion—are tools that educators employ regularly (Figley, 2002). "Compassion is feeling and acting with deep empathy and sorrow for those who suffer" (Hudnall, 2002, p. 107). Sound familiar?

Listening to Others' Trauma Stories Takes a Toll

Jim is a 25-year-old veteran, 5th grade Language Arts teacher working in a school where 85% of the children qualify for free and reduced lunch. He is a good listener and compassionate by nature. He struggles with the sheer volume of stories his students share with him on a daily basis. The chaos of their home lives, the food instability, the exposure to drugs and illegal activities—countless stories that never end. Some days, his mental energy is so depleted because of the day to day psychological wear and tear in which he is experiencing through a series of stages.

Figley's Traumatic Stress Theory (2002) asserts that individuals working directly with others who have been traumatized can be just as likely to experience traumatic stress and related disorders. In other words, you can be traumatized merely by working with and listening to individuals who have a trauma history (Valent, 2002). Upon hearing these trauma stories, secondary traumatic stress can occur. Educators demonstrating resentment, neglect, and distress could be experiencing compassion stress. "The distress and trauma of not having done enough to avert suffering or death is a common secondary stress and secondary trauma response in helpers" (Valent, 2002, p. 26). When your feelings become overwhelming, due to an empathic response to students, your belief systems can be disrupted (Saakvitne & Pearlman, 1996). In 2017, I conducted a qualitative study with 22 pre-service teachers. I asked them to describe the emotions they experienced when dealing with a secondary traumatic incident. Participants were in their senior year of college.

A number of studies have determined that workers who are frequently exposed to traumatized children are *especially* vulnerable and are at a higher risk for developing compassion fatigue (Figley, 2002; Meyers & Cornille, 2002). Chapter 2 discussed the developmental impact of trauma as it relates to child development. Educators are dealing with children who are traumatized, but many also have their own personal histories that can play a role in their perception of a secondary, traumatic event. Briere and Elliot (2003) found that a staggering 76% of American adults have experienced at least one traumatic event. Anda et al. (2006) had similar findings in their seminal ACES study. DuBois (2010) found that two-thirds of the special education teachers working in an early intervention (ages 3–5) program had experienced at least two adverse childhood experiences with several of the participants reporting more.

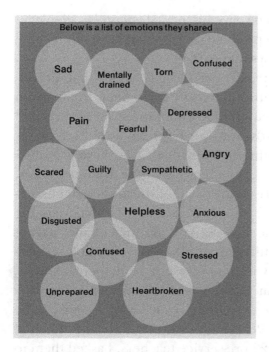

Figure 5.1 **Emotions experienced when dealing with a secondary traumatic incident.**

My mother needed to go on welfare for the first time in her life, needed to go get food stamps. She was left with five children to raise and the youngest has special needs ... [I had personally] experienced the excitement of people passing along bags of used clothing and we would go through the bag and say "I got dibs on this, I got dibs on that." Knowing how valuable just somebody passing along some simple used clothing could be ...

(Female teacher, 23 years' experience)

In this study, the early intervention teachers shared that this impacted the way they interacted with their students and the daily decision-making that took place (DuBois, 2010). These personal experiences can shape not only how the secondary trauma material is processed, but also which coping mechanisms are employed when addressing physiological, psychological, and emotional needs. Research has found that workers with a personal history of trauma are at a greater risk for developing secondary traumatic stress, which ultimately can lead to compassion fatigue if not appropriately mitigated (Figley, 2002; Saakvitne & Pearlman, 1996). As a result, a large number of professionals possess a personal history of traumatic experiences predisposing them to greater risk for long-term issues.

> *Well, my mom was sick whenever I was younger [a small child], and my dad says that she was verbally abusive to me. I don't remember. So I blocked that in somewhere. So that's what I'm wondering if some of the things I'm hearing with the children is some of the things inside of me that are coming out ... He [her father] tells me about it now as an adult ... I feel a lot of compassion for them [the children] because ... I want them to be children ... I can empathize.*
>
> (Female teacher, 12 years' experience)

How Does the Downward Spiral Begin?

Subtle differences exist between burnout and vicarious trauma. When an educator's emotional or systemic resources are limited or if the stress is accumulative and unrelenting, burnout can occur. The onset of burnout is typically gradual. Your traumatic experience is secondary to feelings of being overwhelmed and as a result, your worldview is rarely altered (Trippany, Kress, & Wilcoxson, 2004). There is good news! You can swiftly remediate burnout by making lifestyle changes or altering your current circumstances. It is possible, however, for individuals to experience both burnout and vicarious trauma if not properly addressed in a timely fashion (Trippany et al., 2004). The pre-service teachers reported a variety of feelings when confronted with trauma material including those shown in Figure 5.2.

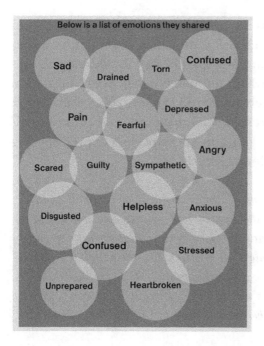

Figure 5.2 **Emotions experienced when confronted with trauma material.**

Secondary Traumatic Stress or Vicarious Trauma?

Empathic engagements are described in the research literature using a variety of terms, ranging from *secondary traumatic stress* (Figley, 2002) to *vicarious traumatization* (Saakvitne & Pearlman, 1996). For the purposes of this book, vicarious traumatization will be viewed as an extension of secondary traumatic stress (Sexton, 1999).

"Vicarious Traumatization is the transformation of the [helper's] inner experience as a result of empathic engagement with ... trauma material ... It is a human consequence of knowing, caring, and facing the reality of trauma" (Saakvitne & Pearlman, 1996, p. 25).

In essence, your cognitive schemas including worldview, identity, psychological needs, beliefs, and memory system are all areas affected when you experience vicarious trauma. These effects can be cumulative and permanent—having an impact on both your professional *and* personal lives (Saakvitne & Pearlman, 1996). The degree of empathy to which you possess can actually exacerbate the impact of vicarious trauma on the individual and could potentially extend to the children in their care (Saakvitne & Pearlman, 1996; Trippany et al., 2004). Essentially, the more compassionate and empathic you are, the higher your risk for developing vicarious trauma. If these negative, destructive behaviors, thoughts, and emotions are not treated, compassion fatigue will occur.

As we move further down this continuum, if neither burnout nor vicarious trauma are properly addressed, compassion fatigue will ensue. Individuals can experience symptoms commensurate with posttraumatic stress disorder.

- Intrusive memories and/or dreams;
- Experience flashbacks;
- Negative self-worth and emotions;
- Detachment and emotional numbness;
- Irritability or aggression;
- Hypervigilance;
- Impaired attention skills;
- Sleep disturbances.

> (taken from APA, 2013, Diagnostic and Statistical
> Manual of Mental Disorders)

Treatment at this point will take time to remediate. Differences in symptomology also exist between vicarious trauma and compassion fatigue. Conversely, Regan et al. (2006) found that individuals exhibiting signs of compassion fatigue demonstrate overt physical symptoms such as exhaustion, impaired functioning, and avoidance/numbing. Put simply, compassion fatigue is the amalgamation of secondary traumatic stress and cumulative burnout experienced by an individual over a period of time (Figley, 2002). Individuals working with children appear to be especially at high risk (Meyers & Cornille, 2002).

What is Compassion Fatigue?

Compassion fatigue can manifest itself in a variety of dimensions, which include: Cognition, Emotional, Behavioral, Spiritual, Relational, Physical, and Professional (Figley, 2002). Warning signs can be evidenced in each dimension helping individuals to identify and address the impact of their lived, professional experiences.

Cognition Takes a Hit

The effect on cognition can take many shapes and the severity can vary day to day. Educators may experience diminished levels of concentration not only when completing work tasks, but also in their personal lives. One male teacher described his experience in this way:

> *I know I was a lot more on edge during [the time when this] was going on. I had a difficult time expressing what needed to be done in the classroom to other people ... I really didn't notice at the time. My spouse mentioned it to me, like a week later: "What's going on? You've been a little more guarded, [a] little different; something's not right, what's going on?" I didn't realize it was affecting me to the point it was. I was just shut down at home. I had a hard time functioning with my children, my spouse. I was there, but I wasn't ... I would say these emotions lasted at least a month and a half, we were on high alert.*

An increase in apathy and disorganization can also contribute to poor work performance, as you care less and less about your students and personal efficacy, in addition to experiencing difficulty organizing all of the moving parts of your life. As work productivity suffers, a decrease in self-esteem can occur as you no longer believe you are effective in their role as a teacher. Dichotomous thinking, or seeing things as *all or nothing* or *black or white*, can occur. This way of thinking can be problematic because it limits your perceived choices and options and can lead to poor decision-making. But wait—there is more! As a component of dichotomous thinking, you can experience a rigidity of thought-processes—*there is only one solution to this issue*—which can also be problematic, especially working in a collaborative environment such as a school. Cognitive disorientation or experiencing confusion in life and work roles and responsibilities can have an impact as well. To the extreme, educators may be experiencing thoughts of self-harm or a desire to hurt others (Figley, 2002). Surprisingly, professionals in this dimension may try to minimize what they are experiencing, thereby denying themselves the opportunity to properly process the gravity of the moment.

Compassion Fatigue Can Bring on the Feels ... or Not

Compassion fatigue can elicit a number of complex emotions. Feelings of anxiety, fear, sadness, and depression are common. Hypersensitivity, common in secondary traumatic stress, can occur as you attempt to visualize and/or process the traumatic event. Educators often report a feeling of powerlessness over their ability to control the traumatic situation. Sound familiar? As a result, you can experience guilt and anger, which can lead to feelings of overall numbness—leading to emotional depletion (Figley, 2002).

> *First sadness and shock that people can be as cruel as they are sometimes. And just, I want children to be children and to think that they can't have a childhood really hurts me ... I feel anger too. How can people do this? How can they just have these beautiful children and treat them like this? ... Fatigue [is another] thing. Because it just seems like when the day is over, it's not over. Because you are either thinking or you are trying to write something to be right for the children ... whenever you are trying so hard to manage the class, and try to take care of some of these things at the same time.*
> (Female teacher, 12 years' experience)

Ch-Ch-Ch-Changes ... Behaviorally

Behaviorally, changes in sleep patterns can be a strong, initial indicator that stressors from work are having an impact on you. Sleep disturbances include getting too little sleep or experiencing an increase in the overall number of hours spent asleep. Nightmares can also manifest at this time. Variances in sleeping patterns can contribute to an increase in irritability, impatience, and moodiness (Figley, 2002). Studies have linked a diminished immune system and poor sleep. Sleep deprivation in humans (there are *a lot* of studies out there involving animals!) can affect your immune cell numbers, function, and cytokine production (Bryant, Trinder, & Curtis, 2004). What are cytokines, you ask? These helpful little proteins regulate our immune and inflammatory responses. Bryant et al. (2004) also found that chronic sleep loss, due to shift work, pressured lifestyles, various stressors, and overall changes in society may be more detrimental to immune function than episodes of short-term total loss.

Sleep disturbance is a big one with me. I have a hard time keeping my brain—I can't turn it off at night. I can lay down and say, "It's time to sleep, it's time to rest," but it doesn't keep the wheels from spinning, and sometimes it will actually manifest in dreams or I'll be thinking, 'What can I do?'

(Female teacher, 10 years' experience)

Sleep gets harder because it gets hard to go to bed at night and put it all to rest. Sometimes I'm just so exhausted that I'll fall asleep, but then I wake up at 3:00am and I keep thinking, "I should keep one of these little recorders [beside my bed]" because my mind starts going into school and doing this, and doing that, and what I need to do, and what I should have done. So then, you're dealing with tiredness, exhaustion, which makes things harder.

(Female teacher, 26 years' experience)

Your appetite can also be profoundly affected. Who's guilty of emotional eating? As it turns out, there are physiological reasons why! Both extremes of the spectrum occur ranging from over-eating as a method of coping to loss of appetite. Maniam and Morris (2012) found that the systems that control both food intake and stress responses *share the same anatomy*! As a result, stress can alter your feeding behaviors with both increases and decreases of food intake observed. The severity of the stress you are experiencing appears to have an overall effect on intake and also predisposes you to seek out energy and nutrient-dense foods (Torres & Nowson, 2007). In other words, when you are feeling overwhelmed, you favor foods rich in sugar and fat.

> *I notice some weight loss or weight gain; it just fluctuates. Sometimes when I'm overstressed, I don't eat at all. Sometimes I'm not thinking, I eat too much.*
> (Female teacher, 10 years' experience)

> *Over-eating is another thing that I do to cope. I can tell when I have a rough day 'cause my ankles are big.*
> (Female teacher, 12 years' experience)

> *I obviously cope too much because I like the sweets!*
> (Female teacher 26 years' experience)

What Am I Doing with My life?

Educators tend to enter the profession because they want to make a difference in the lives of children (DuBois, 2010). Research has found that individuals in caring professions derive tremendous satisfaction in knowing that they have provided quality care and compassion to others, which in turn motivates them to continue on with their work (Stamm, 2002). As compassion fatigue develops, you may begin to question your sense of purpose and life's meaning (*What difference am I making in this child's life? Why did I become a teacher?*). Listening to kids' stories about all of the bad happening to them, forces educators to confront their faith (*How can God let this happen? Is there a God?*). Your spiritual life can be deeply uprooted.

Social Connections, Anyone?

We all experience moments when we need to be alone or take a break from others. The degree to which this happens and the frequency of our withdrawal can be a reasonable gauge on how problematic this behavior is. Schools are (mostly!) a collegial environment. Colleagues notice when previously social co-workers disappear into their offices or classrooms. As educators withdraw from others on a frequent, consistent basis, the danger is that loneliness, isolation, and a lack of intimacy occur (Figley, 2002). As a result, we unknowingly reduce a support system of colleagues who not only understand our lived experiences, but can validate our thoughts and feelings.

> *I say a lot of times, almost an upset stomach or just [dealing with the] anxiety was upsetting. I guess I would just get more upset to my stomach or I wasn't able to eat as much ... just kind of going about [my day] and hoping it would go away.*
>
> (Female teacher, 10 years' experience)

What's Wrong with Me Physically?

Chronic, toxic stress can also have an impact on immunity. We experience stress in a number of ways, including our work environment. If the work burden is accumulative and surpasses our threshold to manage the stress effectively, we have little time to recover and restore our mental and emotional balance. Personally, any major life transition (i.e. marriage, divorce, death of a loved one) creates additional stress. This continuous, unrelenting mental load can impact us neurologically disrupting sleep and daily functioning. Affecting the neuroendocrine-immune network, the toxic stress reaction can lead to an ongoing, abnormal cortisol response (Johnson, Riley, Granger, & Riis, 2013; Wolf, Miller, & Chen, 2008). As a result, the immune system becomes dysregulated, increasing the risk and frequency of infections (Wyman et al., 2007; Caserta et al., 2008; Fagundes, Glaser, & Kiecolt-Glaser, 2013).

Physically, educators can experience an increased heart rate, sweating, and breathing difficulties—separate from or related to panic attacks. Vague aches and pains can also be reported (Figley, 2002). Exhaustion is a common complaint (Figley, 2002).

> *I've certainly noticed an increased heart rate as the time got closer and closer [to the child's coming to school]. I'm sure my blood pressure was up because I was always warm. I just felt like I was racing to get stuff done. And I know I was a lot more on edge during the first part of all of that stuff that was going on … Probably for the first week and a half, it took me a good three hours to fall asleep. I would stay up thinking about what I could've done and I would be up to one or two in the morning, which made it difficult to function at work. I think after that first week and a half, my body was just so exhausted from being up late and getting up early, it had to fall asleep.*
> (Male teacher, 10 years' experience)

> *My stomach—just to keep the stomach acid down because stress levels get crazy.*
> (Female teacher, 26 years' experience)

Am I Losing Touch Professionally?

Having a sense of control can be fundamental in choosing a constructive path when feeling overwhelmed. Control helps us frame a stressful situation into one in which we can take charge and shape our role. Richards (2012) found that an educator's feelings over her lack of control in decision-making was one of the top five contributors of teacher stress. Adding the dimension of secondary trauma, increases this feeling of powerlessness. As a result, overall morale and motivation (personal and school-wide) can be low.

Procrastination, anyone? When we lack motivation, our ability to complete tasks is decreased as we increase our avoidance of completing any undesirable assignments. An overall negativity towards our work, coupled with a detachment to our students can foster a lethal apathy, harmful to the educational process in general. As educator caseloads and overall job responsibilities have increased, so have the needs of students. The constant strain to meet students' needs while fulfilling multiple job roles and maintain compassion and composure can feel immense.

Additional Resources

The ProQOL can be found in Appendix B of this book. www.Proquol.org/uploads/ProQOL_5_English_Self-Score_7_2011.pdf

The link provides a useful tool to enable you to assess your current stress level. www.healthcentral.com/sleep-disorders/stress-test-3454-143.html

"How to manage compassion fatigue in caregiving by Patricia Smith" TED Talk https://www.youtube.com/watch?v=7keppA8XRas

"Deconstructing compassion fatigue by Nikita Amir" TED Talk https://www.youtube.com/watch?v=U_4qIz0jMZU

Self-Reflective Questions for Thoughtful Practice

Self-awareness is critical in properly identifying when you are experiencing distress. The questions below will allow you to examine how you function when experiencing vicarious trauma. Please take a moment to reflect on how your values and beliefs influence your thoughts and behaviors.

When I am confronted with a child's traumatic experience I:

Think:

_____

_____

_____

_____

Feel:

_____

_____

_____

_____

Act:

_____

_____

_____

_____

How do my values and beliefs shape my thoughts, feelings, behaviors?

_____

_____

_____

_____

What is one destructive behavior I should address?

_____

_____

_____

_____

What symptoms of compassion fatigue have I experienced?

_____

_____

_____

_____

How did I address these symptoms?

_____

_____

_____

_____

What interventions worked and/or what would I change about how I addressed these symptoms?

_____

_____

_____

_____

What do I have the power to change?

_____

_____

_____

_____

References

American Psychiatric Association (APA). (2013). *Diagnostic and statistical manual of mental disorders* (5th ed.). Arlington, VA: American Psychiatric Publishing.

Anda, R. F., Felitti, V. J., Walker, J., Whitfield, C. L., Cremner, J. D., Perry, B. D., Dube, S. R., & Giles, W. H. (2006). The enduring effects of abuse and related adverse experiences in childhood: A convergence of evidence from the neurobiology and epidemiology. *European Archives of Psychiatry & Clinical Neurosciences, 256*(3), 174–186.

Briere, J. & Elliot, D. (2003). Prevalence and psychological sequelae of self-reported childhood physical and sexual abuse in a general population sample of men and women *Child Abuse & Neglect, 27*(2003), 1205–1222.

Bryant, P. A., Trinder, J., & Curtis, J. (2004). Sick and tired does sleep have a vital role in the immune system. *Nature Reviews Immunology*, *4*(6), 457–467.

Caserta, M. T., O'Connor, T. G., Wyman P. A., Wang, H., Moynihan, J., Cross, W., Tu, X., Jin, X. (2008). The associations between psychosocial stress and the frequency of illness, and innate and adaptive immune function in children. *Brain Behavioral Immunology*, *22*(6), 933–940.

DuBois, A. L. (2010). *An inquiry into the lived experiences and contextual understandings of early childhood special educators related to children's trauma*. (Doctoral dissertation.) Duquesne University.

Fagundes, C. P., Glaser, R., & Kiecolt-Glaser, J. K. (2013). Stressful early life experiences and immune dysregulation across the lifespan. *Brain Behavioral Immunology*, *27*(1), 8–12.

Figley, C. R. (Ed.) (2002). *Treating compassion fatigue* (1st ed.). New York, NY: Brunner-Routledge.

Hudnall, E. (2002). Measuring compassion satisfaction as well as fatigue: Developmental history of the compassion satisfaction and fatigue test. In C. R. Figley (Ed.). *Treating compassion fatigue* (1st ed., pp. 39–55). New York, NY: Brunner-Routledge.

Jaycox, L. H., Tanielian, T. L., Sharma, P., Morse, L., Clum, G., & Stein, B. D. (2007). Schools' mental health responses after Hurricanes Katrina and Rita. *Psychiatric Services*, *58*(10), 1339–1343.

Johnson, S. B., Riley, A. W., Granger, D. A., Riis, J. (2013). The science of early life toxic stress for pediatric practice and advocacy. *Pediatrics*, *131*(2), 319–327.

Kanter, J. (2007). Compassion fatigue and secondary traumatization: A second look. *Clinical Social Work Journal*, *35*, 289–293.

Lantieri, L. & Nambiar, M. (2004). Sustaining the soul that serves: Healing from within. *Reclaiming Children and Youth*, *13*(2), 120–124.

Maniam, J. & Morris, M. J. (2012). The link between stress and feeding behavior. *Neuropharmacology*, *63*(1), 97–110.

Mathieu, F. (2012). *The compassion fatigue workbook: Creative tools for transforming compassion fatigue and vicarious traumatization*. New York, NY: Routledge.

Meyers, T. & Cornille, T. (2002). The trauma of working with traumatized children. In C. R. Figley (Ed.). *Treating compassion fatigue* (1st ed., pp. 39–55). New York, NY: Brunner-Routledge.

Regan, J., Burley, H. L., Hamer, G., & Wright, A. (2006). Secondary traumatic stress in mental health professionals. *Tennessee Medicine*, 39–40.

Richards, J. (2012). Teacher stress and coping strategies: A national snapshot. *The educational forum*, *76*, 299–316.

Saakvitne, K. W. & Pearlman, L. A. (1996). *Transforming the pain: A workbook on vicarious traumatization*. New York, NY: W. W. Norton & Company.

Sexton, L. (1999). Vicarious traumatisation of counselors and effects on their workplaces. *British Journal of Guidance and Counseling*, *27*(3), 393–403.

Stamm, B. H. (2002). Measuring compassion satisfaction as well as fatigue: Developmental history of the compassion satisfaction and fatigue test. In C. R. Figley (Ed.), *Treating compassion fatigue* (1st ed., pp. 107–119). New York, NY: Brunner-Routledge.

Torres, S. T. & Nowson, C. A. (2007). Relationship between stress, eating behavior, and obesity. *Nutrition*, *23*(11–12), 887–894.

Trippany, R. L., Kress, V. E., & Wilcoxson, S. A. (2004). Preventing vicarious trauma: What counselors should know when working with trauma survivors. *Journal of Counseling and Development*, *82*(1), 31–37.

Valent, P. (2002). Diagnosis and treatment of helper stresses, trauma, and illnesses. In C. R. Figley (Ed.) *Treating compassion fatigue* (1st ed., pp. 17–38). New York, NY: Brunner-Routledge.

Wolf, J. M., Miller, G. E., & Chen, E. (2008). Parent psychological states predict changes in inflammatory markers in children with asthma and healthy children. *Brain Behavioral Immunology*, *22*(4), 433–441.

Wyman P. A., Moynihan J., Eberly S., Cox C., Cross W., Jin X., Caserta M. T. (2007). Association of family stress with natural killer cell activity and the frequency of illnesses in children. *Arch. Pediatr. Adolesc. Med.* (161), 228–234. Retrieved on August 22, 2018 doi: 10.1001/archpedi.161.3.228.

6

COMPASSION SATISFACTION
You're Pretty Darn Awesome!

I have resilience and insight. I know when to get help, when I need it, and try to help others do the same. Sometimes, I am the help.
(Female undergraduate peer educator)

Introduction

Even though the focus of the previous chapter centered on negative outcomes related to trauma exposure, there can be positive outcomes as well. When you are exposed to students' trauma, you have the opportunity to reframe its meaning and grow personally and professionally from the experience. When educators support a child who is dealing with trauma, they can derive tremendous satisfaction in knowing that they have provided quality care and compassion, which in turn motivates them to continue on with their work (Stamm, 2002). Resilient educators also recognize that their experience with trauma enables them to develop important insights about themselves and their ability to help others.

Why is it that some people are negatively impacted by trauma, while others are not? Stamm (2002) asserts that less than 8% of trauma-exposed individuals experience any long-lasting negative effects. One might assume that a person's ability to "self-protect" is strong instinctually. Resilience appears to be a factor in promoting growth and positivity in the face of adversity. Resilience is the ability to physically and mentally adapt to environmental changes (Greene, 2009). It is the difference between someone conceptualizing themselves as a survivor versus a victim. The biggest barrier for educators in developing resilience is a negative environment with unrealistic workloads and an organizational culture that does not support staff (Allee, 2015). The biggest support in the development of resilience is a strong coworker connection.

What is Compassion Satisfaction?

Professional quality of life is the quality you feel in relation to your work as a teacher. Professional quality of life is influenced by both positive and negative aspects of doing one's job. Burnout and compassion fatigue represent negative aspects. Positive aspects would include compassion satisfaction. Compassion satisfaction as it relates to student trauma is the "pleasure you derive from being able to do your work well" (Stamm, 2010). You might feel that it is a pleasure, or even a privilege, to help students in need—particularly as an educator. You may have positive feelings about your colleagues or your ability to promote student learning. You may even feel that your work as an educator contributes to the greater good of society.

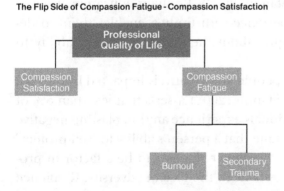

The Flip Side of Compassion Fatigue - Compassion Satisfaction

Figure 6.1 **The flip side of compassion fatigue—compassion satisfaction.**

Rewards of Professional Practice

To examine more closely the nature of compassion satisfaction, it is helpful to reflect on why you became a teacher. In a recent survey, when asked why they chose education as a profession, teachers overwhelmingly spoke of the rewards of teaching (Maier & Phillips, 2013). Not surprising, very few said they chose teaching as a way to make lots of money or to have their summers off. Instead, their answers reflected a passion and commitment to engaging in challenging work.

In total, 98% of the teachers surveyed said they chose teaching in order to make a difference in students' lives. Teachers also spoke about the desire to help students reach their full potential and to make a difference in their schools' community. Serving as an educator is an opportunity to make a difference in an individual student, a specific community, and ultimately, the world.

Teachers also reported wanting to pursue a passion for the craft of teaching. Teaching demands a unique combination of knowledge, skills, and creativity. In total, 74% said they became a teacher to share their love of learning and teaching with others. Two-thirds of the survey respondents (66%) said they became a teacher to experience and be a part of those "aha" moments with students. Half said they became a teacher because a teacher inspired them when they were young.

There is a certain joy that comes from realizing the rewards of teaching. Sometimes this results in a feeling of happiness and satisfaction when you see a student reach a goal you have both worked hard to achieve. Perhaps it is in the form of encouraging words from a colleague when they recognize good things happening in your classroom or with a particular student. These are things that give you energy and motivate you to continue to push forward, even when it is hard. This energy can be fed through good memories of past success, enjoyable work experiences in the present, or positive anticipation of reaping the rewards of teaching in the future.

Essentially, the giver in the helping relationship gets a lot from the giving. Skovholt (1974) identifies four ways that giving can be rewarding. First, the giving role provides an educator with a sense of identity. For many, their identity as an educator includes the need to be effective in their role and feel connected with others in the process. Second, giving is rewarding in that it allows educators to exchange their professional services for other meaningful resources, such as status and appreciation. Third, teachers are rewarded through giving by observing and learning from their students. As an educator, I have learned as much from my students as they may have learned from me. Last, teachers find satisfaction through direct reinforcements. This is often manifested through the approval and affection of students, as well as from their parents and the larger community.

Through our work as educators, we can achieve a certain level of immortality. We are the ones contributing to the ongoing evolution of society. By educating students, we allow them to stand on the shoulders of giants, enabling them to discover and solve mysteries of the universe. Our futures will be better due to their contributions. Investing ourselves in the growth and development of students can provide enormous meaning for an educator. When that meaning seems to disappear, as in the case of burnout, it can be very distressing and it will seem difficult for educators to regain.

Post-Traumatic Growth and Vicarious Resilience

Richard Tedeschi and Lawrence Calhoun (1995) introduced the term *post-traumatic growth* to describe the positive changes that some trauma survivors report as a result of the struggle to cope with traumatic events. Researchers began to wonder if those positive changes extend to the helper as well. Termed *vicarious post-traumatic growth*, those who are exposed to trauma by helping others can also experience positive changes in the areas of their self-perception, interpersonal relationships, and philosophy of life (Hyatt-Burkhart, 2014).

Vicarious resilience is a phenomenon characterized by "a unique and positive effect" that transforms helpers in response to a trauma survivors' own resiliency (Acevedo & Hernandez-Wolfe, 2014, p. 474). Since teachers and students exist in a shared relationship where they mutually influence each other, it is possible that teachers working with students who experience the trauma of poverty, abuse, neglect, and other forms of adverse experiences are positively impacted through the observation of their students overcoming adversity. One study showed the variety of ways in which vicarious resilience can help teachers make positive meaning of their experience in working with traumatized students (Acevedo & Hernandez-Wolfe, 2014). Those positive effects included:

- *Affect regulation as a relational activity.* Teachers found that by developing a teaching relationship based on trust, consistency, and empathy, they could better connect with their students. As students opened up, teachers developed the skills that allowed them to hear their students' stories calmly and compassionately. Students who previously demonstrated in negative behaviors were able to mimic and adopt teacher behavioral cues, creating a culture in the classroom that positively affected other students.
- *Expansion of relational skills.* Teachers found that focusing on the cognitive aspects of the classroom without attending to the emotional needs of their students made classroom management difficult. Focusing on relational aspects with students, which at times meant a departure from the daily schedule or curriculum, opened a space for students to reflect on and articulate their experiences in a variety of mediums. Relational skills were also expanded in regard to making connections with students' families to extend the goals of the classroom into the home.
- *Resonance with own adversities.* For some teachers, students' experiences provided an opportunity to reflect on their own personal adversities. Seeing the process of helping

their students overcome adversity as a relational experience, teachers reflected on their commitment to develop
meaningful relationships with their students and accepted
their responsibility to take additional steps to help students
in need.

- *Changes in interpersonal relationships.* After much experience in
  working with students who had experienced trauma, teachers reported changes in their own approach to interpersonal
  relationships. Some reported becoming more compassionate, others saw themselves as being more effective as parents,
  and others found the strength to expect more in their own
  personal relationships.
- *Reassessment of one's problems.* Observing the challenges and
  adversities their students faced enabled teachers to take a different perspective on their own problems. When comparing
  their problems to that of their students, teachers described
  an approach to life where they complained less, felt stronger
  in the face of adversity, and lived their life happier.
- *The impact of trauma and constructivist learning strategies.*
  Teachers learned that they had to change and adjust their
  approach to the classroom to accept and work with each student's needs. Pedagogically, this meant adopting learning
  approaches that permitted and encouraged students to connect their personal experiences with the curriculum. Writing
  exercises were effective for student self-expression, and a variety of readings were effective in exposing students to other
  experiences and perspectives.
- *Perspective-taking and flexibility.* Teachers discussed how being exposed to the trauma of their students influenced their
  desire to learn more about their students and their lived
  contexts. They developed a greater understanding of the
  complexities of their students' lives and in doing so, felt better prepared to address the obstacles to learning their students face. Teachers also discussed how their perspective
  shifted. Instead of approaching their students from a deficit-
  based approach, they developed an appreciation for the
  inherent strengths of their students. This shift was further

aided by a more flexible perspective, which allowed them to be more adaptive and responsive to student needs.

- *Recognition and affirmation of racial and gender identity diversity.* As teachers became more aware of abuse and the negative impact it has on students, they became more responsive to both victims and perpetrators. Addressing these issues also raised teacher awareness of the issues surrounding racial, sexual, and gender identity.
- *Raising critical consciousness and advocacy.* Teachers became more outspoken regarding the obstacles their students faced. They saw it as their responsibility to talk about social issues affecting their students to positively influence educational policy and resource allocation.

These positive outcomes for teachers working with students who have experienced trauma help to highlight the many ways post-traumatic growth can occur. These teachers experienced vicarious resilience by developing new ways of thinking and acting as a result of witnessing their students overcome adversity. Hopefully, these examples of vicarious resilience can assist you in shifting your perspective as it relates to working with students who have experienced trauma.

Developing and Sustaining Compassion Satisfaction

When educators are able to develop and sustain compassion satisfaction, they are more likely to stay in the profession and remain effective in their work. To maintain an enthusiasm for the field of education, we need to experience compassion satisfaction on a regular basis. Developing and sustaining compassion satisfaction involves engaging in activities that increase our positive outlook. Three ways of doing so include keeping a positive attitude towards students, increasing opportunities to manage stress, and implementing meaningful self-care (Radey & Figley, 2007). There are many steps that you can take to maximize these three avenues to develop and maintain a positive outlook.

There are several ways educators can maintain a positive attitude towards students. This can be supported through a positive work environment and appropriate venues to discuss student issues and successes. Workload variety provides educators with a broader platform to experience student success. Also, a manageable workload and appropriate time off, as well as drawing healthy boundaries between work and personal life will help educators to develop and sustain compassion satisfaction.

Educators can manage stress through access to physical, intellectual, and social resources. These resources are critical in developing and sustaining compassion satisfaction. In addition to teacher training, access to meaningful professional development will assist teachers in expanding their intellectual resources. Teachers should be able to reach out to others, building a supportive network of colleagues, friends, and family.

Meaningful self-care is also necessary for educators to maintain a connection with the rewards of their work. Satisfaction with one's role as a helper to students experiencing trauma can only occur if the helper themselves is in a healthy physical and mental state. Proper nutrition, regular exercise, and adequate sleep can blunt the body's physical and hormonal reactions to stress, which contributes to improved mood and thinking (Silverman & Deuster, 2014). A positive mental state enables you to better experience the rewards to helping students, and see yourself as an effective caregiver in your role.

What aspects of your role as an educator give you the most satisfaction? For some, they take great satisfaction from their work in helping students learn and grow. Others may get lots of pleasure from their work with colleagues or their ability to contribute to an overall positive school environment. The satisfaction you derive from your job can come from a variety of sources, and impact you in different ways.

How Do I Know if I am Experiencing Compassion Satisfaction?

Another way to assess whether you are experiencing compassion satisfaction is using the *Professional Quality of Life Scale* (ProQOL) located in Appendix B at the back of this book.

The ProQOL measures negative and positive aspects of being a helper using three sub-scales: burnout, compassion satisfaction, and compassion fatigue. Higher scores on the compassion satisfaction sub-section of the ProQOL means that you experience greater satisfaction as it relates to your ability to be an effective educator.

Additional Resources

Saenz, A. L. (2011). *The power of a teacher.* Peoria, AZ: Intermedia Publishing Group, Inc. A TED Talk presented by Adam is available at this web address: https://www.youtube.com/watch?v=AyogyD7vXbw
    Smith, P. (2012). *Compassion satisfaction: 50 steps to healthy caregiving.* Healthy Caregiving, LLC.

Self-Reflective Questions for Thoughtful Practice

Compassion satisfaction keeps your batteries charged, and helps combat the development of burnout and compassion fatigue. It is important to celebrate victories (however small!) and reconnect with the reasons why you chose to become an educator. Use the following questions to reflect on your "why," and explore the ways you can boost your sense of compassion satisfaction.

Why did you choose to become an educator?

_____

_____

_____

_____

What specific experiences have made you feel rewarded as an educator?

_____

_____

_____

_____

What specific experiences have you had that enabled you to see yourself or your students in a new way?

_____

_____

_____

_____

What are some ways you can increase the number of positive work experiences that feed your energy for your work?

_____

_____

_____

_____

References

Acevedo, V. E., & Hernandez-Wolfe, P. (2014). Vicarious resilience: An exploration of teachers and children's resilience in highly challenging social contexts. *Journal of Aggression, Maltreatment & Trauma, 23*(5), 473–493.

Allee, A. (2015). *Resilience: Mid-level student affairs professionals' lived experiences* (Doctoral dissertation).

Greene, R. R. (2009). Risk and resilience theory: A social work perspective. In R. R. Greene (Ed.), *Human behavior theory & social work practice* (3rd ed., pp. 315–434). Piscataway, NJ: Aldine Transaction.

Hyatt-Burkhart, D. (2014). The experience of vicarious posttraumatic growth in mental health workers. *Journal of Loss and Trauma, 19*, 1–10.

Maier, M., & Phillips, V. L. (2013). *Primary sources: America's teacher on teaching in an era of change.* New York, NY: Scholastic, Inc. and Bill & Melinda Gates Foundation.

Radey, M., & Figley, C. R. (2007). The social psychology of compassion. *Clinical Social Work Journal, 35*(3), 207–214.

Silverman, M. N., & Deuster, P. A. (2014). Biological mechanisms underlying the role of physical fitness in health and resilience. *Interface focus, 4*(5), 20140040.

Skovholt, T. M. (1974). The client as helper: A means to promote personal growth. *The Counseling Psychologist, 4*(3), 56–64.

Stamm, B. H. (2002). Measuring compassion satisfaction as well as fatigue: Developmental history of the compassion satisfaction and fatigue test. In C. R. Figley (Ed.), *Treating compassion fatigue* (pp. 107–119). New York, NY: Brunner-Routledge.

Stamm, B. H. (2010). *The Concise ProQOL Manual* (2nd ed.). Pocatello, ID: ProQOL.org.

Tedeschi, R. G., & Calhoun, L. G. (1995). *Trauma and transformation.* Thousand Oaks, CA: Sage Publications, Inc.

7

FOLLOW THE YELLOW BRICK ROAD ... TO RECOVERY!

When the well's dry we know the worth of water.
                                                    Benjamin Franklin

Educators form strong bonds with the children in their care. Through training and even institutional support, little is done to insulate them from experiencing pain and anguish upon hearing a child's trauma story. Educators must employ compassion when dealing with families who are struggling in their parenting practices and with children who are exhibiting extreme behavioral needs. Possessing a positive affect can influence other important resources needed for self-care. Strong self-care enables us to access our social resources, make better decisions, and experience a more positive overall and effective functioning level. Positivity can expand our scope of thoughts and actions because it allows us to explore, cooperate, and interact with others. As a result, we are better equipped to exercise broader cognitive flexibility and be more creative with addressing our needs (Radey & Figley, 2007). Our life experiences inform the inner resources we access in times of distress. Therefore, interventions must be considered with great care. Several of the techniques recommended in this chapter are well established in fields like counseling and social work, however, these strategies are also effective if implemented consistently within the field of education. Prevention is a key element in addressing burnout and compassion fatigue. Taking a proactive approach can stave off the potential for secondary trauma to have a significant impact later.

Yassen (1995) posits that there are three levels of prevention: primary, secondary, and tertiary. The first layer of prevention encompasses education, awareness workshops and trainings, and self-care plans. The secondary level includes support groups, supervision, and consultation services. The last level involves more specific interventions such as debriefings and personal therapy. In Chapter 5, I talked about a research study I had conducted with pre-service teachers. One of the questions I asked gauged the types of coping mechanisms that they employed when feeling burned out. Here are examples of their responses:

Constructive:

- Spending time with friends;
- Writing/journaling;
- Exercise;
- Spending time outdoors;
- Praying/Spirituality;
- Talking to loved ones;
- Reading;
- Listening to music;
- Removing themselves from the situation.

Destructive:

- TV binge-watching;
- Excessive sleeping;
- Comfort eating;
- Shopping ("retail therapy");
- Isolation.

The Critical Role of Self-Awareness

Self-awareness is an important self-protective behavior and can help us maintain a healthy balance of empathy (Saakvitne & Pearlman, 1996). Poor self-awareness can limit our ability to accurately identify signs of personal distress quickly and remediate them effectively. Understanding our strengths and weaknesses, how our belief system impacts decision-making, and our own perception of self-efficacy can play a critical role in how we address work stressors. Being able to take a critical, hard look at one's self is a crucial first step. It enables us to more firmly decide when to seek help or support. We also open ourselves up to more possibilities to learn and grow through reading, supervision, and professional development experiences. Helping others to learn and develop awareness about the signs and symptoms of burnout and compassion fatigue is also paramount in prevention.

Boundaries

The role of empathy plays a large part in an educator's professional efficacy. Empathy allows individuals to show compassion to not only their students, but also colleagues, who are struggling with life's daily demands. Having compassion for families who are struggling in their parenting practices and demonstrating patience with the children in their care are critical elements in a classroom.

Kathy is a veteran teacher with over 17 years' experience. She grew up in a household with a single parent making minimum wage and multiple siblings. When she has students in her class that demonstrate a similar profile, she often finds herself buying clothes and groceries for the family. Sound familiar? When educators blur boundaries with the children and families in their care, the damage can affect not only their physical selves, but their psyches as well. This hurt can accumulate and be long-lasting. Some educators put up a "shield that keeps [them] at arm's length away," but this only disassociates them from the pain. The implementation of healthy boundaries can be critical in allowing the educator to maintain their psychic and physical selves. Boundaries can allow the educator to create a healthy distance from the pain their student is experiencing. The successful implementation of boundaries extends through many layers of an individual's professional life. Boundaries ensure that a separation exists between the individual and their work. Maintaining regular work hours, taking periodic breaks throughout the day, maintaining a manageable workload are just a few examples to promote balance.

> *I've gone home crying ... It just rips a hole in my heart so big. That is always difficult—leaving this nucleus to go home. You have got to learn to leave what goes on in the child's home in their home because you can't change that. There is nothing I can do that is going to make [their home] better.*
>
> (Female teacher, 19 years' experience)

Self-Care Plans

Another effective preventative strategy is a self-care plan. These plans address specific strategies and behaviors that educators can employ while coping with the roles and responsibilities of their job. The beauty of a self-care plan is that it compels us to *proactively* create constructive actions and behaviors to engage in during times of stress, in addition to crisis planning when traumatic situations occur. In essence, self-care plans help us engage in self-reflection by identifying positive aspects of our lives that can be accessed during times of distress. These plans can include a number of elements, however, most address goals in each of the areas shown in Figure 7.1.

Examples of a physical support might be incorporating exercise into the day, eating healthy, or getting enough sleep at night. Staff have incorporated this in a number of ways including creating a group who walks the track at lunchtime, providing a physical and social outlet in the middle of the day. Psychological supports could include taking a break from technology, seeking effective supervision, or keeping a reflective journal. Emotional care can include focusing on positive aspects of the day such as engaging in a hobby with friends or having a confidant with whom to vent. Spiritual supports may involve engaging in mindfulness or meditative practices and attending church/mosque/or temple. Attending special events and nurturing close relationships

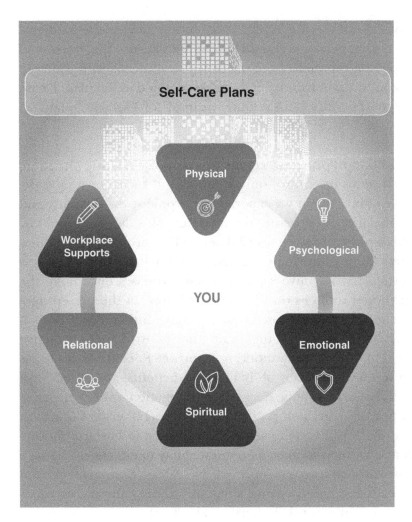

Figure 7.1 Self-care plans.

can maintain relational supports. Engaging in professional development and maintaining boundaries can serve as workplace supports on a self-care plan. In an educational setting, this practice also provides administrative personnel with an additional layer of accountability, as they would have tangible behavioral goals that could be activated when the worker is experiencing distress due to the nature of their job. Self-care plans can be adapted to fit the needs of the institution and/or the nature of the work. Supervisors should take care to ensure that personnel completing the plans have the access and means with which to carry out the behavioral benchmarks outlined in the plan. Please refer to Appendix D for another example of a self-care plan.

Mindfulness

Being mindful provides "cognitive" space to fine-tune our attention. It helps us control our attention and focus for longer periods of time. When we experience chronic stress and burnout, an imbalance is occurring between our job's demands and our mental/physical resources (Bakker, & Demerouti, 2007). Mindfulness helps individuals regulate emotional states that possess a particularly negative valence. These exercises encourage the practitioner to focus on the "here and now" of the present moment and stay on purpose in an accepting and kind way (Kabat-Zinn, 2003). Areas of the brain that control focus, salience detection, and mind-wandering improve. Recent research has uncovered a number of behavioral benefits associated with mindfulness including decreased rumination over a negative situation and greater positive emotions (Luberto, Cotton, & McLeish, 2012). Coping self-efficacy, rooted in Eastern philosophy and defined as one's perceived ability to effectively manage stressors, encourages a more passive rather than active action when addressing a negative situation, thereby increasing one's perception of control (Luberto et al., 2012).

Mindfulness-based Interventions (MBIs) encompass two key features: the ability to focus one's attention and to harness one's orientation to curiosity and openness (Sharp & Jennings, 2016). Mindfulness training can improve areas of the brain assisting in learning, cognition, memory and emotional regulation as well as increases in positive attitude, self-compassion, gratitude, and empathy (Shapiro, Brown, & Biegel, 2007). Training in this area can ultimately decrease anxiety and stress. It helps to prevent us from evaluating and judging ourselves and creates an open space for us to learn and develop. By reframing the positive, we can bring our negative thoughts and emotions under control.

Professionals who participate in MBIs report reductions in somatic symptoms, stress, burnout, and negative mood (Abenavoli et al., 2013). Spirituality can serve as a significant protective factor as it affects the way a person perceives hope and life meaning (Saakvitne & Pearlman, 1996). Spirituality also fosters connections among individuals. The research findings of Luberto et al. (2012) suggest that "the mindfulness skill of accepting without Judgment may improve emotion regulation by promoting self-efficacy for coping with stressors" (p. 163).

Visualization can also be a powerful tool. Visualization exercises should focus on positive feelings and be grounded in your own personal real-life experiences. These exercises can allow you to focus on overcoming a fear, achieve personal insight over a particular anxiety you are experiencing, or improve your focus to pursue a meaningful goal.

Everyone Has a Story

Gladding (2016) has said that "writing enables self-expression, acceptance of feelings, and sometimes an increase in one's sense of spirituality" (p. 137). The creation of a story can be transformative. We use stories each and every day to shape our lived experiences. Words help us to inform, connect, share and process. By sharing our thoughts, feelings, and experiences, we are using words to make meaning and find our sense of purpose. Human beings are socially wired and our reality is constructed as such. In other words, the way we experience others is influenced by our perception of these verbal and non-verbal interactions. Words can have power and if we harness it to help make sense of our experiences, healing and growing can occur.

Narrative techniques were first introduced in the 1980s by David Epston and Michael White (1992). The basic premise posits that within the context of an individual's values, culture, and social environment, a person's story can prove fundamental in evaluating their thoughts and behaviors (Metcalfe, 2017). Individuals are asked to write a description of themselves and redefine who they are based on their value system and who they want to be. What Epston and White (1992) call "redescription" compels the person to free themselves of existing labels or stigmas ("the anorexic," for example) and create a new vision of themselves to feel empowered. Every aspect of a person's life—self-perception, description of the problem, values, ideal life—is defined using the individual's own language. The first step in the process is to describe how the individual presents themselves to the world. By viewing life in "chapters," one can begin to unpack a variety of events—some successful, some not—in an effort to focus on *gaps* in their problem story, or exceptions, when the individual presented their ideal version of themselves to the world. At this stage, the individual is identifying their values, beliefs, and strengths and acknowledging the exceptions to the problem. By viewing our lives in *chapters*, we can externalize the problem to view it as an outsider, creating a space to acknowledge our role in the problem. This stage leads to an understanding of how a ripple effect is created. Throughout the process, key words are recorded and used when discussing achievements in other aspects of life and highlighting the skills employed to achieve them. Lastly, the individual will generate a new concept of self and stronger relationships. A fundamental tenet of narrative techniques is the presence of hope exists to remind the person that the struggle does not have to continue indefinitely. They can take control of their narrative over and over again. Pennebaker as stated in Gladding (2016) asserts that journaling about topics that are meaningful can improve an individual's physical and emotional well-being just as much as talking about an individual's trauma experience. Please refer to Appendix E for examples of Narrative techniques.

Exercise Your Funny Bone

Humor activates our sense of spontaneity and pleasure because it actively forces us to engage mentally and physically with others. Gladding (2016) states,

> *Humor, particularly when accompanied by laughter, creates physiological, psychological and social changes. The skeletal muscles become more relaxed, breathing changes, and the brain releases endorphins.*
>
> (p. 185)

Humor allows us to create distance from our current problem or situation and begin to view it from a different perspective. This allows us to change distressing emotional states and perception of a negative emotion or experience and re-frame our thought process or the way we are viewing our current circumstances or environment. Humor also allows us to become more self-aware so that we can better assess what can be done to reduce our anxiety and be less judgmental of ourselves. It enables us to connect with others. Implementing humor can be a slippery slope, however, and administrators and mentors should be mindful of the tone used. If there is an undercurrent that is angry or cynical, an intervention is warranted. If the joke removes the child or family's dignity, it can change or shape the educator's views about those individuals in detrimental and demeaning ways. Humor that is responsible, respectful, and relatable is appropriate. It enables us to reduce the psychological power a traumatic situation can have on us and help us to connect with others in similar experiences. Having a sense of humor also allows us to relieve pent up emotional conflicts and can even relieve depression (Sultanoff, 2003). Having a sense of humor enables us to build up a psychological buffer against our worst days and have transformative effects. Some days if you don't laugh, all you will do is cry!

The Call of Nature

The benefits of exercise have long been reported. There is a growing body of research that has been looking at the effects of *green exercise*—that is, exercise in a natural environment (Flowers, Freeman, & Gladwell, 2018). Spending time in natural settings helps us regulate states of emotional and physiological arousal, reduce negative effects, and increase our feelings of pleasure (Duvall, 2010).

The evidence indicates that nature can make positive contributions to our health, help us recover from pre-existing stresses or problems, have an "immunizing" effect by protecting us from future stresses, and help us concentrate and think more clearly (Pretty, Peacock, Sellens, & Griffin, 2005).

Getting out amongst the trees appears to have a positive effect on our blood pressure, self-esteem, and mood (Rogerson, Brown, Sandercock, Wooller, & Barton, 2016; Anderson & Brice, 2011)!

When Exposed to Trauma, Utilize the Four Quadrant Model

There are ways to help educators initiate self-care planning; one such way is described by Middleton (2015). Divided into four quadrants, this framework explores possibilities for self-care before, during, right after, and later/ongoing when working with individuals who have experienced trauma. It is important for educators to be aware of their own reactions to trauma, and to intentionally adopt resiliency strategies within all four quadrants. However, Middleton (2015) noted that many professionals are only able to identify the activities they can do to practice good self-care for the later/ongoing quadrant. This model can assist educators in developing resiliency habits appropriate for first three quadrants.

Before educators are exposed to the trauma of others, they should engage in good self-care. This includes getting good sleep and eating something nutritious before beginning the work day. Educators should develop activities that transition them into the work environment. This might include getting a cup of coffee or tea to start the work day, taking a few minutes to review your schedule for the day to mentally "prep" yourself, and doing a grounding self "check-in." For a grounding self "check-in," a professional might ask themselves the following questions: (1) How am I feeling today? (2) What is my goal for today? and (3) Who can support me in case I need it? Lastly, when working with students who have experienced trauma, educators should be aware of, and have worked through their own history of trauma. A well-prepared educator is able to be present and attuned to the needs of their students.

While an educator is responding to student trauma, self-care strategies are crucial to successful trauma integration. *During* that time, the educator should focus on the task at hand, stay attuned and grounded, and maintain awareness of their physical responses to the situation, such as breathing, posture, and body awareness. It is important to limit imagery as the student is telling their story. Educators should try to focus on facts, and refrain from playing the story like a movie in their head. The use of mantras—a statement repeated frequently to reinforce a basic belief—can be helpful as well. Professionals can use mantras to remind themselves that it is possible to "help others without having to live their pain" (Middleton, 2015, p. 6).

Right after experiencing secondary trauma is a good time to engage in relaxation and movement. Deep breathing can help slow the heart, reducing blood pressure. Visualization exercises help to clear the mind, allowing a person to transition out of the stressful environment. Movement, such as a short walk through the hallways, can move a person physically out of a stressful space. Walking, stretching, and basic tai chi or yoga movements can also bump up the production of endorphins, which promotes feelings of well-being.

Self-care on a *later/ongoing* basis after exposure to students' traumatic material should involve working with a supervisor or colleagues to debrief the experience. When debriefing, it is important to keep in mind that it should be a structured, intentional conversation, reflecting on professional performance in working with that particular student. Other resilience strategies appropriate for the later/ongoing quadrant include incorporating practices for spiritual renewal and focusing on the satisfaction that comes along with performing a difficult helping role well.

Appendix C provides a visual means of thinking about how to build resilience into your daily practices at work, and specifically when you are confronted with a students' trauma. The Four Quadrant Model can assist you in ensuring that you are engaging in self-care practices before, during and after being exposed to traumatic material.

Organizational and Systemic Responses to Burnout and Compassion Fatigue

Not only is there a personal cost for those suffering from burnout and compassion fatigue, but there are costs to organizations as well. When educators suffer from burnout and compassion fatigue, districts can incur costs associated with absenteeism, loss of productivity, and increased healthcare costs (Stahl, 2016). It is estimated that at least one million people per day miss work because of stress-related issues (Kosinski, 2014). This can account for up to 60 percent of employee absences, which costs employers an average of $602 per individual per year. Therefore, it is in the interest of districts and administrators to mitigate the negative effects of stress on educators.

The personal and organizational costs of burnout and compassion fatigue have led to many proposals for addressing these concerns among workers. Some organizations might intervene when burnout occurs, while others focus on how to prevent stress-related concerns by promoting employee satisfaction and resilience. Approaches to prevent burnout and compassion fatigue among educators can happen at the individual, work group, school, or district levels. In general, the primary focus has been on individual strategies, despite the research evidence that many of the conditions that promote compassion fatigue and burnout occur at the organizational level (Maslach & Leiter, 2016). The remainder of this chapter will explore how improved environmental conditions and certain administrative actions can assist districts in creating more supportive working conditions for educators.

Environmental Conditions in the Workplace

Behavior results from the interaction between the person and the environment (Lewin, 1936). These behaviors serve to produce the environmental culture, which can be described as the collection of assumptions, beliefs, and values that an educator uses to understand the meaning of events and actions in the workplace (Schein, 1992). The perception by educators regarding how they are supposed to respond to stress and student trauma will influence their behavior in either a positive or negative manner, depending on the messages they receive within the workplace (Strange & Banning, 2015). Schools lacking a supportive work environment in regard to the effects of stress and student trauma will increase the likelihood of educators engaging in behaviors that promote the development of burnout and compassion fatigue. Educators and their work environment should be envisioned as an ecosystem, where any change in the environment is reflected in a change in the work experience (Kaiser, 1975). Therefore, implementing strategies to improve the work environment will serve to create a healthier work experience for educators.

- *Reduce negativity in the workplace.* One of the biggest environmental problems can be the cynicism and negativity of co-workers (Mathieu, 2012). Sometimes this takes the form of "bitching, moaning, and whining" (p. 73) about many aspects of the job. Other times it can take the form of mistrust, complaining about upper administration, parents, or the larger community. When you begin to sense you are continually getting the short end of the stick as an educator, you can lose your belief that you have any ability to make any positive contributions as a teacher. Surround yourself with others who are willing to decline participation in negative talk associated with the job. Remember, positive interactions with your co-workers are associated with increased perception of job satisfaction!
- *Leadership needs to set an example regarding self-care.* Leaders within an organization strongly influence the culture by setting an example of attitudes and behaviors that are acceptable in that environment. Leadership sets a positive example for self-care by working a sustainable and reasonable pace over time, and encouraging staff in the district to do the same. Leadership should openly value things and people outside of work. This may include time spent with family,

as well as personal activities and hobbies. Acknowledge that work in the education field can be challenging, and that self-care takes practice and intentionality.

- *Promote social connections, build in humor and fun.* As discussed earlier in this book, social connections are one the protective factors in warding off burnout and compassion fatigue. School environments should encourage social connections, boost morale, and promote positive working relationships. This can be accomplished by ensuring educators develop positive and productive work teams, which can help ensure that no educator is feeling isolated from other co-workers. Seek out opportunities for staff to engage in social activities in the school and outside of it as well. Put together a team that coordinates "fun." Establishing peer support networks within a school or district can also provide opportunities for educators to connect with each other, both formally and informally, which can be helpful for educators when coping with difficult work situations (Boyle et al., 2012).

Organizational Actions

Beyond strategies to improve the work environment, districts can assess whether there are appropriate working conditions, policies, and supports that can mitigate the effects of burnout and compassion fatigue. Some of these are basic considerations for staff. Do staff have adequate salary and balanced workloads? Is there sufficient orientation, professional development, and administrative supervision to ensure educators feel competent and supported in their jobs? Do educators in the district have access to medical and mental health support services? And more importantly, are they encouraged to avail themselves of those services when necessary? Other strategies districts should implement are as follows:

- *Provide positive staff support.* Leadership within the district and individual buildings should adopt strategies to ensure staff feel supported and valued. Encourage communication and staff contributions. Make sure that teachers have voice in decision-making. Take time to collect and integrate teacher feedback to improve learning or services within the district. Leadership should educate staff on how decisions are made, especially in regard to resource allocations, policies, and work assignments. Try to build task diversity and job enrichment into the work. Ensure staff have opportunities for adequate breaks during work.

- *Demonstrate appreciation for staff.* Praise and acknowledge effort and results whenever possible. Educators want to know that they matter, and administrative support extends beyond the jobs that they do. Express concern for the general well-being of the staff in the district. While the quality of the work they do is important, staff wellness should be a foundational concern. Staff well-being directly impacts their productivity and effectiveness in working with students.

- *Promote awareness regarding burnout and compassion fatigue.* Every time we give presentations to educators on the topics of burnout and compassion fatigue, participants are immediately engaged. They recognize that what they are experiencing has a name and it is a REAL THING! Until that point, they had thought they were failing as educators, and are relieved to find that what they are feeling is normal given the demands placed upon them. A common question that gets asked is, "Why aren't we talking about this in my building, or learning about it during a professional in-service?" Acknowledging that educators can develop burnout and compassion fatigue normalizes the experience, and educating staff about it helps to raise awareness around the conditions that promote its development. Beyond education on these topics, school or district leadership should not say or do things that would stigmatize staff who are struggling with secondary trauma or other stress-related issues.

- *Effective supervision of staff.* Provide support for educators affected by the emotional impact of working with students. Be alert to how the cumulative exposure to stressful and traumatic situations may be affecting educators in the district. Regularly check in with staff to see how they are coping. Do not wait for them to approach administrative leadership regarding burnout and compassion fatigue.

- *Establish debriefing processes.* School systems should develop debriefing practices for use by educators encountering traumatic material in the course of their work with students. Debriefing plays an important role in assisting educators to reflect on the skills they employed while working with students who have experienced trauma. Debriefing can also be used as a strategy to mitigate the negative effects of secondary trauma. Instead of "informal" debriefing with friends, family and colleagues, where the tendency is to share all of the graphic details, Mathieu (2012) recommends low-impact debriefing. In low-impact debriefing, the graphic details are kept to a minimum, and the focus is on the individual and organizational response to the student. This ensures that traumatic material shared in consultation with an administrator or fellow colleague does not cause further stress to either party. Refer to Appendix G for specific details regarding how to engage in low-impact debriefing.

- *During times of increased pressure or stress, help staff keep challenges in perspective.* Remind staff of the mission of the school or district. Help them to see how their work fits into that bigger picture. Remind staff of the value the district and community places on them as people and as staff. Educators are the district's most valuable resource! Encourage the development of strategies for staff to work in sustainable ways. When dealing with student crises, help staff strategize how they might use healthy ways of combating stress.

Hopefully, this chapter has helped you to think about specific steps you can take to promote a healthier, more resilient YOU. Increased resilience will enable you to more effectively deal with the stressors associated with your professional role. Like any habit, these methods will take time and effort to integrate into your lifestyle and professional practice. However, the effort is worth the results.

Additional Resources

Morgan, A. (2000). *What is narrative therapy: An easy to read introduction*. Dulwich Centre Publications. Adelaide, Australia.

White, M. (2007). *Maps of narrative practice*. New York, NY: W. W. Norton & Co.

The following is a link to the website of the Traumatology Institute. This site provides resources for dealing with trauma in the schools, as well as an online program to earn School Trauma Certification. http://psychink.com/ticlearn/ti-goes-online/about-us/

Self-Reflective Questions for Thoughtful Practice

Taking time out of your day to engage in self-care can be a challenge. This chapter discussed a number of ways to pause and reflect on what you are experiencing. Answer the questions thoughtfully below, then try out a few of the exercises outlined in the chapter.

How would those who know you intimately describe you on your best days?

_____

_____

_____

_____

On a scale of 1–10, where would you rate your level of self-awareness? Name two strategies you could use to improve your self-awareness.

_____

_____

_____

_____

What are the things your school or district already does well to support educators who are supporting students who have experienced trauma?

_____

_____

_____

_____

References

Abenavoli, R., Jennings, P., Greenberg, M., Harris, A., & Katz, D. (2013). The protective effects of mindfulness against burnout among educators. *The Psychological Education Review, 37*(2), 57–69.

Anderson, R. J., & Brice, S. (2011). The mood-enhancing benefits of exercise: Memory biases augment the effect. *Psychology of Sport and Exercise, 12*(2), 79–82.

Bakker, A. B., and Demerouti, E. (2007). The job demands-resources model: State of the art. *Journal. ManagementPsychology, 22,* 309–328. doi: 10.1108/02683940710733115

Boyle, C., Topping, K., Jindal-Snape, D., & Norwich, B. (2012). The importance of peer-support for teaching staff when including children with special educational needs. *School Psychology International, 33*(2), 167–184.

Duvall, J. (2010). Enhancing the benefits of outdoor walking with cognitive engagement strategies. *Journal of Environmental Psychology, 31,* 27–35.

Epston, D. & White, M. (1992). *Experience, contradiction, narrative & imagination: Selected papers of David Epston & Michael White 1989–1991.* Adelaide: Dulwich Centre Publications.

Flowers, E. P., Freeman, P. and Gladwell, V. F. (2018). Enhancing the acute psychological benefits of green exercise: An investigation of expectancy effects. *Psychology of Sport and Exercise, 39*, 213–221.

Gladding, S. (2016). *The creative arts in counseling* (5th ed.). ACA.

Kabat-Zinn, J. (2003). Mindfulness-based interventions in context: Past, present, and future. *Clinical Psychology Scientific Practice, 10*, 144–156. doi: 10.1093/clipsy.bpg016

Kaiser, L. R. (1975). Designing campus environments. *NASPA Journal, 13*(1), 33–39.

Kosinski, M. (2014, September 25). The cost of career burnout, and how to handle it. Retrieved from https://www.recruiter.com/i/how-to-avoid-career-burnout/

Lewin, K. (1936). *Principles of topological psychology*. New York, NY: McGraw-Hill.

Luberto, C., Cotton, S., & McLeish, A. (2012). Mindfulness and emotional regulation: The mediating role of coping self-efficacy. *Complementary and Alternative Medicine, 12*, 163.

Maslach, C., & Leiter, M. P. (2016). Understanding the burnout experience: recent research and its implications for psychiatry. *World Psychiatry: Official Journal of the World Psychiatric Association (WPA), 15*(2), 103–111.

Mathieu, F. (2012). *The compassion fatigue workbook: Creative tools for transforming compassion fatigue and vicarious traumatization*. New York, NY: Routledge.

Metcalfe, L. (2017). *Solution-focused narrative therapy*. New York, NY: Springer Publishing Co.

Middleton, J. (2015). Addressing secondary trauma and compassion fatigue in work with older veterans: An ethical imperative. *Journal of Aging Life Care, 5*, 1–8.

Pretty, J., Peacock, J., Sellens, M., & Griffin, M. (2005). The mental and physical health outcomes of green exercise. *International Journal of Environmental Health Research, 15*(5), 319–337.

Radey, M. & Figley, C. (2007). The social psychology of compassion. *Clinical Social Work, 35*, 207–214.

Rogerson, M., Brown, D. K., Sandercock, G., Wooller, J. J., & Barton, J. (2016). A comparison of four typical green exercise environments and prediction of psychological health outcomes. *Perspect Public Health, 136*(3), 171–180.

Saakvitne, K. W. & Pearlman, L. A. (1996). *Transforming the pain: A workbook on vicarious traumatization.* New York, NY: W. W. Norton & Company.

Schein, E. H. (1992). *Organizational culture and leadership.* (2nd ed.) San Francisco, CA: Jossey-Bass.

Shapiro, S., Warren Brown, K., & Biegel, G. (2007). Teaching self-care to care-givers: Effects of mindfulness-based stress reduction on the mental health therapists in training. *Training and Education in Professional Psychology, 1*(2), 105–115.

Sharp, J. & Jennings, P. (2016). Strengthening teacher presence through mindfulness: What educators say about the cultivating awareness and resilience in education (CARE) program. *Mindfulness.* V.7, (1), 209–218.

Stahl, A. (2016, March). Here's what burnout costs you. *Forbes.* Retrieved from https://www.forbes.com/sites/ashleystahl/2016/03/04/heres-what-burnout-costs-you/#12c2ab8c4e05

Strange, C. C., & Banning, J. H. (2015). *Designing for learning: Creating campus learning environments for student success* (2nd ed.). San Francisco, CA: Jossey-Bass.

Sultanoff, S. (2003). In C. Schaefer (Ed.). *Play therapy for adults.* (1st ed. pp. 107–143). New Jersey, Wiley & Sons.

Yassen, J. (1995). Preventing secondary traumatic stress disorder. In C. R. Figley (Ed.), *Compassion fatigue: Coping with secondary traumatic stress disorder in those who treat the traumatized.* (pp. 178–208). New York: Brunner/Mazel.

APPENDIX A

Assessing Risk Factors that Contribute to the Development of Burnout and Compassion Fatigue

There are many ways you can assess which factors might put you at risk for developing burnout and compassion fatigue. We have compiled a series of questions that you may find useful in assessing your risk factors. Take some time to reflect on the following elements that correspond to the nature of your work environment, the nature of your professional role, the nature of the individual, and the nature of the broader social context. Consider to what extent you feel distress regarding any of the following.

The school environment:
- What events, incidents, cases, circumstances are the most difficult? Why?
- How much control do you have over your schedule?
- Does this schedule work for you? Can you adequately negotiate your workload?
- How has the workload changed over the years?
- Do your work tasks vary from day to day?
- Do you like the work you do?
- Are you sufficiently trained to do the work you do?
- How much support do you have?
- Is supervision adequate, helpful, supportive?

Your professional role as an educator:
- Is your work as an educator personally fulfilling?
- Is your workload manageable? How would you describe the quality and quantity of your workload?

- Do you have variety regarding the types of students you work with?
- What types of students are the most difficult for you and why?
- How do your students treat you? Are you ever afraid of your students?
- Have you ever been harmed by a student?
- How do you treat your students?

Your individual needs:
- How well suited are you personally for the work you do?
- How well does the work you do match your values and beliefs?
- How stressed are you? Can you identify the factors in your life that produce the most stress?
- What is your own experience with trauma? How does this impact your work and overall well-being?
- What coping mechanisms do you use to manage or decrease stress?
- Do you have supportive interpersonal relationships?
- Do you engage in a hobby or leisure activity every week?
- Do you have healthy coping strategies?

Nature of the social/cultural context:
- What are the social obstacles to doing your work? (funding cuts, workload, etc.)
- How are you received within the community based on the work that you do and the work of your organization?
- Do you feel the work you do is respected?
- What does the community say about the students you serve?
- What effect, if any, does the above have upon you personally?

Bibliography

Mathieu, F. (2012). *The compassion fatigue workbook: Creative tools for transforming compassion fatigue and vicarious traumatization.* New York, NY: Routledge.

Saakvitne, K. W., Pearlman, L. A., & Abrahamson, D. J. (1996). *Transforming the pain: A workbook on vicarious traumatization.* New York: WW Norton.

APPENDIX B
The Professional Quality of Life (ProQOL) Survey

Beth Stamm (2010) and Charles Figley have done extensive research on the relationships between burnout, compassion fatigue, and compassion satisfaction. In doing so, they have developed a self-test called the ProQOL (Professional Quality of Life). This test can be used free of charge to assess your own levels of secondary trauma, burnout and compassion satisfaction. The ProQOL has been used and studied widely across many different helping professions, and is considered to be a highly reliable and valid measure of the costs of helping others.

There are two ways you can take the ProQOL. It is reproduced on the following pages. You can also download copies of this survey at http://www.proqol.org/ProQol_Test.html. On the survey, you may substitute "teacher" or "educator' for the term [helper] in each of the items. When you have completed the ProQOL, you can calculate your scores. Be sure to follow the directions provided for scoring for the burnout subscale. It is scored a bit differently than the other two subscales.

It is important to recognize that the ProQOL is not a diagnostic test. Burnout, secondary traumatic stress, and compassion satisfaction are not official mental health diagnoses. If you are experiencing symptoms of depression and/or anxiety, it is best to explore those issues with a mental health professional.

For more information about the history of the ProQOL, taking the survey, and interpreting the results, refer to the *ProQOL Concise Manual* (2nd ed.) at https://proqol.org/ProQOl_Test_Manuals.html.

Professional Quality of Life Scale (ProQOL)

Compassion Satisfaction and Compassion Fatigue
(ProQOL) Version 5 (2009)

When you *[help]* people you have direct contact with their lives. As you may have found, your compassion for those you *[help]* can affect you in positive and negative ways. Below are some-questions about your experiences, both positive and negative, as a *[helper]*. Consider each of the following questions about you and your current work situation. Select the number that honestly reflects how frequently you experienced these things in the *last 30 days*.

1=Never	2=Rarely	3=Sometimes	4=Often	5=Very Often

_____ 1. I am happy.
_____ 2. I am preoccupied with more than one person I *[help]*.
_____ 3. I get satisfaction from being able to *[help]* people.
_____ 4. I feel connected to others.
_____ 5. I jump or am startled by unexpected sounds.
_____ 6. I feel invigorated after working with those I *[help]*.
_____ 7. I find it difficult to separate my personal life from my life as a *[helper]*.
_____ 8. I am not as productive at work because I am losing sleep over traumatic experiences of a person I *[help]*.
_____ 9. I think that I might have been affected by the traumatic stress of those I *[help]*.
_____ 10. I feel trapped by my job as a *[helper]*.
_____ 11. Because of my *[helping]*, I have felt "on edge" about various things.
_____ 12. I like my work as a *[helper]*.
_____ 13. I feel depressed because of the traumatic experiences of the people I *[help]*.
_____ 14. I feel as though I am experiencing the trauma of someone I have *[helped]*.
_____ 15. I have beliefs that sustain me.
_____ 16. I am pleased with how I am able to keep up with *[helping]* techniques and protocols.
_____ 17. I am the person I always wanted to be.
_____ 18. My work makes me feel satisfied.
_____ 19. I feel worn out because of my work as a *[helper]*.
_____ 20. I have happy thoughts and feelings about those I *[help]* and how I could help them.
_____ 21. I feel overwhelmed because my case [work] load seems endless.
_____ 22. I believe I can make a difference through my work.
_____ 23. I avoid certain activities or situations because they remind me of frightening experiences of the people I *[help]*.
_____ 24. I am proud of what I can do to *[help]*.
_____ 25. As a result of my *[helping]*, I have intrusive, frightening thoughts.
_____ 26. I feel "bogged down" by the system.
_____ 27. I have thoughts that I am a "success" as a *[helper]*.
_____ 28. I can't recall important parts of my work with trauma victims.
_____ 29. I am a very caring person.
_____ 30. I am happy that I chose to do this work.

Figure B.1 **Professional Quality of Life Scale (ProQOL).**

Reference

Stamm, B. H. (2010). *The concise ProQOL manual* (2nd ed.). Pocatello, ID: ProQOL.org.

APPENDIX C
The Four Quadrant Model of Trauma Self-Care

Table C.1

The Four Quadrant Model of Trauma Self-Care

Before	During
• Engage in consistent physical and emotional self-care • Transitions to work • Transitions to trauma • Recognize and anticipate triggers	• Focus on the task at hand • Stay present and grounded • Breath, posture, and body awareness • Create distance or protection: a space around yourself, a step back, take a moment • Use of mantras • Limit imagery • Notice your reactions and plan to examine those later • Leave the trauma when you leave

Later/Ongoing	Right After
• Body awareness: relaxation or movement techniques • Breathing exercises • Visualization exercises • Stay connected to others, avoid isolation • Transitions from trauma • Transitions from work	• Regular practice of relaxation techniques and/or physical movement or exercise • Build and use broad professional and social support • Take care of your physical and emotional health • Develop interests and activities outside of work

Bibliography

Middleton, J. (2015). Addressing secondary trauma and compassion fatigue in work with older veterans: An ethical imperative. *Journal of Ageing Life Care, 5*, 1–8.

APPENDIX D
Mindfulness Exercises

Releasing Negative Emotions

1. Lie down. Close your eyes.
2. Take three deep breaths.
3. The first minute is spent on answering the question, "how am I doing right now?" while focusing on the feelings, thoughts and any bodily sensations that arise and trying to give these words and phrases.
4. The second minute is spent on keeping awareness on the breath.
5. The third minute is used for an expansion of attention from solely focusing on the breath, feeling the ins and outs and how they affect the rest of the body.
6. Now focus on an emotion that is troubling you or you have a difficult time controlling. Is it anger, frustration, anxiety? Only think about that emotion. What does it feel like?
7. As you breathe in, imagine you are gaining strength and as you exhale-imagine you are releasing that emotion and its negative energy.
8. Continue breathing in and gaining strength. Exhaling and releasing the negativity.
9. Find a natural pattern to your breathing.
10. When you're ready slowly open your eyes.

Strengths and Weaknesses

1. Lie down and close your eyes.
2. Find a steady rhythm to your breathing.

3. Now breathe deeply in for four counts, then exhale through your nose. Repeat four times.
4. Clear all thoughts from your mind.
5. Today we're going to focus our thoughts on our strengths and weaknesses.
6. Great humans possess intimate knowledge of both. Your strengths are already bearing fruit. We often tend to address only our strengths. Improving the weight that we bench. Earning a starting position on the team. Improving our grades. Are your strengths academic? Athletic? Social? Are you kind? Generous? Patient? Do you set a strong example? Are you mentally tough? Are you a good leader?
7. Continue to breathe.
8. Now examine your weaknesses. A more abundant future is waiting for you if you are in touch with your weaknesses and work on making them strengths. We often neglect acknowledging our weaknesses and as a result, do not perform at our optimum. Do you lack discipline? Do you lack focus or follow through? Are you a poor listener? Are your relationships unfulfilling?
9. Imagine a bright light entering your body at the top of your head. This light is connecting you with the power to embrace your weaknesses today and grow stronger. Let this light wash over your neck, shoulders, chest, abdomen, legs, and feet. Do you have clarity on what you will work on today? The power is within you to do so.
10. Continue to breathe and as you concentrate only on this task, reassure yourself with the knowledge that you have strength to endure the challenges set before you.
11. Take three more deep breaths and when you're ready, open your eyes.

APPENDIX E
Narrative Technique

Statement of Position Map

This simple handout consists of three areas to be filled in:

1. Characteristics and naming or labeling of the problem.
2. Mapping the effects of the problem throughout each domain of life it touches (home, work, school, relationships, etc.).
3. Evaluation of the effects of the problem in these domains.

Values that come up when thinking about these effects are undesirable. This map is intended to be filled out in concert with a therapist, but it could be explored individually if it is difficult to find or meet with a narrative therapist.

Generally, the dialogue between a therapist and client will delve into these three areas. The therapist will ask questions and probe for deeper inquiry, while the client talks through the problem they are having and finds insight into each of the three main areas listed above.

There is power in the simple act of naming the problem, and it is necessary to understand how and in which areas the problem is having an effect. Finally, it is vital for the client to understand why this problem bothers them on a deeper level. What values are being infringed upon or obstructed by this problem? Why does the client feel negatively about the problem? These are questions that this exercise can help to answer.

Retrieved from https://positivepsychology.com/narrative-therapy/on April 15, 2019.

Strategies for Promoting Positive Emotions

Anchoring: An outside stimulus that activates a positive inner state or reaction within you (i.e. Memory of a favorite person or place).

Touchstone triggering: Anchoring exercise in which you carry a small object that you associate with happiness.

Implementation of slogans or quotes: Identify slogans or quotes that inspire you and put you in a positive frame of mind. Use as wallpaper on your phone or post on your desk.

What will I do tomorrow: At the end of each day, identify three achievable tasks that you can accomplish the next day. The idea behind this is rooted in the concept that "success breeds success".

Thought stopping: Identify a situation that you always associate with negative thoughts or emotions. Identify the negative statement that you make when this occurs. Take some deep, purposeful breaths. Then say a phrase that cues you to stop your negative thoughts.

Bibliography

Strycharczyk, D. & Clough, P. (2015). *Developing mental toughness: Coaching strategies to improve performance, resilience, and well-being.* London: Kogan Page Publisher.

APPENDIX F
Self-Care Plan Diagram

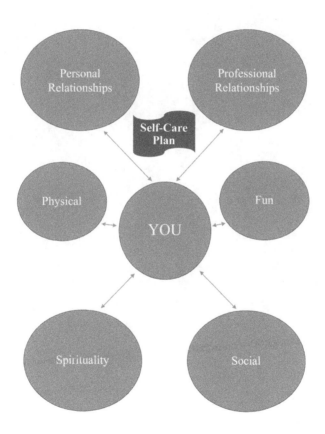

APPENDIX G
Retelling a Student's Story
Low-Impact Debriefing Strategies

They say it is helpful to talk about the things that bother you. But is it healthy to repeat over and over the traumatic details associated with one of your students? Instead of storytelling with friends, family and colleagues, where the tendency is to share all of the graphic details, Mathieu (2012) recommends low-impact debriefing. Debriefing is a way of talking about your interaction with a student who has experienced trauma. A structured debriefing with a supervisor or colleague can assist you in dealing with the physical or psychological symptoms that are generally associated with trauma exposure. Debriefing also provides you the opportunity to process the event and reflect on its impact. Low-impact debriefing involves four key steps to ensure what traumatic material is shared in consultation with a supervisor or fellow colleague does not cause further stress to either party. The first step involves increased self-awareness. Think through the following questions:

- What are the ways you debrief with others?
- How much detail do you share?
- How much detail do others share with you?
- How do you best deal with traumatic material?

The second step involves fair warning. People are better able to accept and respond to traumatic material if they know beforehand they will be receiving it. Schedule time to debrief with another person, or if the need to discuss the incident is more urgent, be sure to provide advance notice before launching into a description of the story. Related to fair warning is the third step—consent. After giving fair warning, be sure to obtain consent before you share. This gives the listener a chance to decline or to confirm what they are able and ready to hear. In this scenario, a teacher might approach their principal or school counselor and say, "I just met with a student who is struggling with a difficult situation. Is this a good time to talk?" Your colleague might respond with, "I have a little time now. Can you share without going into lots of detail?"

The fourth and last step focuses on limited disclosure. Mathieu (2012) recommends starting from the outside of the story with the least traumatic information, and moving gradually towards the core, where the most traumatic material resides. Sometimes sharing graphic details is necessary. However, evaluate if sharing, and how much, of the traumatic material is necessary for a professional discussion focusing on how to best address the needs of the student. Additionally, how much traumatic material needs to be shared with another for self-evaluation purposes? Minimizing exposure (and re-exposure) to traumatic material is an important strategy for keeping educators healthy.

Reference

Mathieu, F. (2012). *The compassion fatigue workbook: Creative tools for transforming compassion fatigue and vicarious traumatization.* New York, NY: Routledge.

INDEX

103; staff supervision 103–104; support during pressured times 104; supporting work environment: positive self-care examples by leadership 101–102/promotion social connections 102/reduced negativity in workplace 101; *see also* administrative teaching support, quality of

personal characteristics as source of burnout 46–47; demographic characteristics (sex, age, race, education, marital/family situation) 46t; personality characteristics (self-concept, needs, motivations, emotional control) 47t
professional quality of life: burnout 78f; compassion fatigue 78f; compassion satisfaction 78f; secondary trauma 78f; *see also* *Professional Quality of Life Scale* (ProQOL)
Professional Quality of Life Scale (ProQOL), as burnout indicator 54, 84–85
professional support, quality and availability of: 33–36, 41; involved/detached supervisor 33–36; *see also* teacher attrition; self-efficacy; compassion stress/fatigue, risks factors

recovery from compassion fatigue, burnout 89–105; setting boundaries 91–92; exercise in nature 97–98; humor 96–97; mindfulness 94–95; prevention, three levels of 89–90; self-awareness 90–91; self-care plans 92–94, 93f; *see also* Four-Quadrant Model of trauma self-care 95–96

resilience/vicarious resilience 6; to grow compassion satisfaction 6, 77, 80–83; positive and negative influence on 78, Four-Quadrant Model of trauma self-care 99, *see also* organizational and systematic responses to burnout, compassion fatigue

self-efficacy: and administrative support 33–36; and job-continuation rates 6; and resilience 6; *see also* burnout; compassion stress/fatigue
sense of ineffectiveness/inadequacy, symptoms of: apathy 52; increased irritability 52; lack of productivity/poor performance 52; *see also* burnout, symptoms
socio-economic background, and experience abuse, violence 15, 16, 33
Spradley, James P. 52–54
Stamm, Beth H. 6–7, 77
stress/anxiety, definition 21

teaching as job: educational and personal demands 2; psychological preparedness 2
teacher attrition: coping-affecting factors (external/internal) 4–5; professional support, quality and availability of 33; role of administrative/collegial support 4; trauma and 4–7; trauma training, lack of 31; *see also* administrative teaching support, availability and quality of
teacher training, lack of trauma preparedness in teacher training 2, 11, 29–32, 84, 89; as source of burnout and

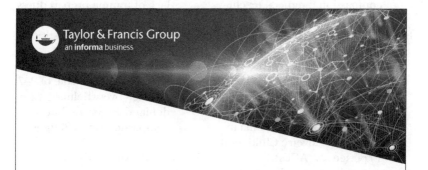